# Global Primary Mental Health Care

This book provides up-to-date, practical information for family doctors on how to assess and manage important mental health problems presenting in primary care settings.

Patients frequently present with mental health problems in primary care settings around the world, yet family doctors consistently identify gaps in their knowledge, skills and confidence in how best to care for them. Contributors to the book are experts in primary mental health care and have consulted with family doctors around the world, to identify their main learning needs. Each of the nine core chapters will begin with a set of key points on 'how to do it' and will end with educational material in the form of clinical scenarios and multiple choice questions. This book describes core competencies for primary mental health care, clarifies how to conduct a first consultation about depression, reviews non-drug interventions for common mental health problems, discusses the management of unexplained physical symptoms, and advises on the physical health care of patients with severe mental illness. It explores the mental health needs of migrants and young people, and explains how to manage problems of frailty, multimorbidity and dementia.

This book will be of interest to family doctors and students specialising in family medicine worldwide.

**Christopher Dowrick** is Professor of Primary Medical Care at the University of Liverpool, UK.

# Global Primary Mental Health Care

## Practical Guidance for Family Doctors

*Edited by Christopher Dowrick*

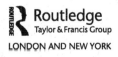

**Routledge**
Taylor & Francis Group

LONDON AND NEW YORK

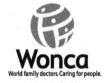

**Wonca**
World family doctors. Caring for people.

First published 2020
by Routledge
2 Park Square, Milton Park, Abingdon, Oxon OX14 4RN

and by Routledge
52 Vanderbilt Avenue, New York, NY 10017

*Routledge is an imprint of the Taylor & Francis Group, an informa business*

*British Library Cataloguing-in-Publication Data*
A catalogue record for this book is available from the British Library

*Library of Congress Cataloging-in-Publication Data*
A catalog record has been requested for this book

ISBN: 978-0-367-13422-8 (hbk)
ISBN: 978-0-367-13424-2 (pbk)
ISBN: 978-0-429-02638-6 (ebk)

Typeset in Univers
by Swales & Willis, Exeter, Devon, UK

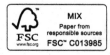

Printed in the United Kingdom
by Henry Ling Limited

# Contents

# Illustrations

## Figures

## Tables

# Contributors

**Bruce Arroll,** Professor of General Practice and Primary Health Care, University of Auckland, New Zealand.

**Weng Yee Chin,** Assistant Professor, Department of Family Medicine and Primary Care, University of Hong Kong, Hong Kong.

**David Clarke,** Assistant Director, Center for Ethics, and Clinical Assistant Professor in Gastroenterology, Oregon Health & Science University, Oregon, USA.

**Alan Cohen,** retired GP, former Director of Primary Care, West London Mental Health Trust, UK.

**Christopher Dowrick,** Professor of Primary Medical Care, University of Liverpool, UK; Chair of Working Party for Mental Health, World Organisation of Family Doctors (WONCA).

**Sandra Fortes,** Associate Professor of Medical Psychology and Mental Health, School of Medical Sciences, State University of Rio de Janeiro, Brazil.

**Marientina Gotsis,** Research Associate Professor, Creative Media and Behavioral Health Center, Interactive Media and Games Division, School of Cinematic Arts, University of Southern California, USA.

**Kim Griswold,** Professor of Family Medicine, Psychiatry, and Public Health and the Health Professions, Department of Family Medicine, Jacobs School of Medicine & Biomedical Sciences, Buffalo, New York, USA.

**Cindy L K Lam,** P Danny DB Ho Professor in Family Medicine and Head, Department of Family Medicine and Primary Care, University of Hong Kong, Hong Kong.

**Christos Lionis,** Professor of General Practice and Primary Health Care, Clinic of Social and Family Medicine, School of Medicine, University of Crete, Greece.

**Fiona Moir,** Senior Lecturer, Department of General Practice and Primary Health Care, University of Auckland, New Zealand.

**Vicki Mount,** GP registrar Auckland Region, New Zealand.

**Maria van den Muijsenbergh,** General Practitioner, Professor of Health Disparities and Person-centered Primary Care, Radboud University Medical Center, Nijmegen; and Pharos, Dutch Centre of Expertise on Health Disparities, Utrecht, the Netherlands.

**Tim olde Hartman,** Associate Principal Investigator, Department of Primary and Community Care, Radboud University Medical Center, Nijmegen, the Netherlands.

**Ferdinando Petrazzuoli,** General Practitioner in Italy, Postdoctoral Researcher, Family Medicine and Community Medicine, Lund University, Sweden.

**Jane Roberts,** GP Partner, Aintree Park Group Practice, Liverpool, UK; former Royal College of General Practitioners Youth Mental Health Clinical Champion.

**Jinan Usta,** Associate Professor, Family Medicine Department, American University of Beirut, Lebanon; President WONCA Eastern Mediterranean Region.

**Venetia Young,** retired GP and safeguarding lead, Cumbria, UK.

# Acknowledgements

We are grateful to the following people for their contributions to the World Organisation of Family Doctors (WONCA) guidance documents and for reviewing new material for this book:

Michael Duncan (Brazil), Jane Gunn (Australia), Amanda Howe (UK), Gabriel Ivbijaro (UK), Ray Mendez (USA), Juan Mendive (Spain), Stewart Mercer (UK), Donald Nease (USA), Aaron Poppleton (UK), Pramendra Prasad (Nepal), Sonia Roache-Barker (Trinidad & Tobago), Louise Robinson (UK), Samuel Wong (Hong Kong) and Chuan Zou (China).

# Preface

Patients frequently present with mental health problems in primary care settings around the world, yet family doctors consistently identify gaps in their knowledge, skills and confidence in how best to care for them. The aim of the book is to provide up-to-date, practical information for family doctors on how to assess and manage important mental health problems presenting in primary care settings.

Depression is now the leading cause of disability. In 2015 there were over 300 million cases of depression worldwide (about 4.4% of the world's population), and the global cost of the disorder was more than one trillion US dollars. The number of people with common mental disorders is increasing, particularly in lower income countries, because the population is growing and more people are living to an age when depression and anxiety most commonly occur.[1]

There is a substantial treatment gap for depression. In low and lower middle income countries, less than 15% of people with a depressive disorder receive any evidence-based treatment for that disorder. In higher middle income and high income countries the situation is not much better, with only between 20% and 30% being offered an effective treatment.[2]

The integration of mental health in primary care is an international priority. Family medicine is well placed to provide effective patient care close to home.[3] However, many family doctors do not currently have sufficient knowledge and skills to give them confidence in caring for patients with common mental health problems. In an assessment of educational needs carried out by the World Organisation of Family Doctors (WONCA) in 2017, mental health was identified by 32% of family doctors in the Asia Pacific region as a priority; it was the most frequently desired area for education.[4]

The World Health Organisation (WHO) has invested considerable time and effort in bridging the treatment gap for depression and other mental health problems. They have identified an impressive range of evidence-based interventions that can realistically be scaled-up in low and middle income countries. The WHO 'mhGAP Intervention Guide', now in its second iteration,[5] provides clear and practical guidance on the assessment and management of the variety of mental health and neurological problems encountered in primary care settings. These include depression, psychoses, epilepsy, child and adolescent mental and behavioural disorders, dementia, disorders due to substance misuse, and self-harm and suicide.

# Scope and structure

This book is intended to support and contribute to the WHO mhGAP programme, specifically by meeting the current expressed educational needs of family doctors.

The scope of the material presented in the book is based on problems identified as important by members of the WONCA Working Party for Mental Health (WWPMH). We have consulted with family doctors around the world, to identify their main learning needs.

This book is a practical 'how to do it' guide for family doctors around the world, enabling them to meet the mental health needs of their patients. It is written by a group of very experienced family doctors, who have a comprehensive understanding of current challenges and how to address them. Each of the core chapters is produced by a small international task group composed of WWPMH members, chaired by the first or named author, in consultation with stakeholders and experts within and beyond WWPMH. They are all based on the latest available evidence, and represent consensus positions on current best practice in global family medicine.

We begin by identifying a set of core competencies for family doctors in primary mental health care working in any part of the world, and indicating how these can be achieved. In Chapter 2 we explain how to conduct the first consultation with a patient presenting with depression. In Chapter 3 we describe a variety of psychosocial and behavioural interventions which can be offered by family doctors for patients with common mental health problems such as anxiety and depression. Then, in Chapter 4, we discuss the assessment and management of patients presenting with unexplained physical symptoms. In Chapter 5 we focus on the physical health care of patients with severe mental illness. Then we consider the mental health needs of migrants in Chapter 6. Chapters 7 to 9 cover mental health problems occurring across the life course, first exploring the needs of young people and then turning to the problems of frailty, multimorbidity and dementia, which are all more common in old age.

Each chapter starts with a summary of key points. We then provide up-to-date, evidence-based practical information for family doctors on how to assess and care for their patients presenting with these problems in primary care settings. We offer educational material, in the form of case studies and multiple choice questions, so that readers can check their own knowledge and skills based on the information we provide. Each chapter concludes with a list of resources for further study, and a set of references.

# Orientation

While we adopt many Western concepts of mental health and disorder, we are mindful that these have their limitations. Experiences of pain and depression, for example, raise questions about assumed distinctions between mind and body. Different cultures have different understandings of the causes and meaning of disorder, and have different expressions or idioms of distress. This is important for family doctors when thinking about possible presentations of depression, or about the presence of unexplained physical symptoms, especially when working in low and middle income countries, or in consultations with recent migrants to high income countries.

While we share concerns about the substantial treatment gap for depression, we do not wish to ignore problems of over-diagnosis and over-medication, particularly in high income countries.[6] Hence we encourage careful and considered approaches to diagnosis, and recommend non-drug interventions wherever possible.

While we promote the importance of accurate diagnosis, we also note the potential for primary care doctors to engage in simple case formulation. It is not sufficient to focus on diagnostic thresholds or duration and severity of symptoms. It is also important to take account of impairment and disability, of social and cultural factors, and of our patients' value systems and cultural beliefs.

While making best use of our own knowledge and skills, we should pay careful attention to our patients' perspectives on what may be causing their problems, not least because these may be radically different from our own. We should be sensitive when elucidating our patients' health beliefs, and enquiring about the ways in which they make sense of their experiences.

As family doctors, what we seek to do in our encounters with patients with mental health problems is to help them to find meaning and purpose out of suffering and distress. This is the essence of healing. At the heart of this process lie two assumptions. The first assumption is that the emergence of meaning, order or form is therapeutic in itself, particularly for people who are feeling lost, alone, frightened or misunderstood. The second assumption is that such emergence is most effective if it is mutual, if we find ways of engaging with our patients' conceptual worlds, if understanding of problems and their solutions are negotiated and agreed by both sides, not just imposed arbitrarily by the doctor.[7]

It may also be instructive to reflect on our basic understanding of our patients. We often assume they are passive victims of disease or circumstance. This may sometimes be so, but by no means always. Instead, we may more profitably see our patients as persons with agency,[8] experts in leading their lives, who sometimes need our help, new ways of looking at old ideas, and perhaps an instillation of hope for the future.

Christopher Dowrick

## References

1. World Health Organisation. Depression and other common mental disorders: global health estimates. Geneva, 2017.
2. Chisholm D, Sweeny K, Sheehan P, et al. Scaling-up treatment of depression and anxiety: a global return on investment analysis. *Lancet Psychiatry.* 2016, 3: 415–424.
3. World Health Organisation and World Organisation of Family Doctors. Integrating mental health into primary care: a global perspective. Geneva, 2008.
4. Kumar P, Larrison C, Rodrigues SB, McKeithen T. Assessment of general practitioners' needs and barriers in primary health care delivery in Asia Pacific region. *J Family Med Prim Care.* 2019, 8: 1106–1111.
5. World Health Organisation. mhGAP intervention guide 2.0. Geneva, 2016.
6. Dowrick C, Frances A. Medicalising unhappiness: new classification of depression risks more patients being put on drug treatment from which they will not benefit. *BMJ.* 2013, 347: f7140.
7. Dowrick C. *Beyond depression,* 2nd edition. Oxford: Oxford University Press, 2009.
8. Dowrick C. Patients, persons, selves. In Dowrick C (ed) *Person-centred primary care: searching for the self.* Abingdon: Routledge, 2018.

Chapter 1

# CORE COMPETENCIES OF FAMILY DOCTORS IN PRIMARY MENTAL HEALTH CARE

Christopher Dowrick and Cindy L K Lam

In this chapter we indicate what can reasonably be expected of all trained and qualified family doctors, working in primary care settings in any part of the world, when caring for people with mental health problems.

# Key points

We consider that there are six domains for the core competencies of family doctors in primary mental health care.

1. **Values:** Family doctors consider mental health to be important.
2. **Communication skills:** Family doctors adopt person-centred approaches to assess, manage and support people with mental health problems.
3. **Assessment:** Family doctors identify and diagnose common mental health problems, and can identify severe mental health problems and assess risk.
4. **Management:** Family doctors manage people with common mental health problems, and the physical health of people with severe mental health problems.
5. **Collaboration and referral:** Family doctors use a range of available options and resources for the care of people with mental health problems, and tailor them to patients' and carers' needs.
6. **Reflective practice:** Family doctors take care of their own health and well-being.

# Introduction

As discussed in the Preface, family doctors see many patients with mental health problems but often do not know how best to help them. In this chapter we provide a set of standards of good practice for family doctors in primary mental health care. We describe the core competencies; what is reasonable to expect family doctors to know and to do when caring for patients with mental health problems.

The core competencies set out in this chapter are based on a consensus of opinion from experienced family doctors from all parts of the world, and from experts from other disciplines. We began with an initial draft set of competencies, which were circulated for comment to all members of the WONCA Working Party for Mental Health (WWPMH). A revised draft was then circulated and received further comments from the World Health Organisation's Department of Mental Health and Substance Abuse, the World Psychiatric Association, the World Federation for Mental Health, the International Association for Communication in Healthcare, and the Royal College of General Practitioners. The final version was approved by the WONCA Executive Committee.

We present the core competencies for family doctors within six domains, and note competencies that are expected for more advanced practice. We offer practical examples, and consider the implications of these competencies for service delivery. We then provide a case study and some multiple choices questions, so you can check your own knowledge and understanding. Finally, we offer a variety of written and online resources for those who would like to learn more.

**1. Values:** Family doctors consider mental health to be important.

Before we start caring for patients with mental health problems, it is important to reflect on our own attitudes towards mental health.

Many family doctors may feel uncertain or anxious about mental health problems, fearing they do not know enough about them, and worrying they will be overwhelmed and unable to cope. This book will help to address these concerns.

Some family doctors may have negative or stigmatising views about mental illness, seeing it as shameful, self-induced, an unnecessary waste of the doctor's valuable time. We strongly disagree with such views. They are the opposite of the values we need.

---

**Core competencies**

- Family doctors treat mental and physical health as of equal importance.
- Family doctors treat patients with mental health problems with dignity and respect.
- Family doctors take responsibility for diagnosing and managing patients with mental health problems, and supporting their families.

---

**Examples**

You take one patient's expression of suicidal ideas just as seriously as the next patient's presentation with chest pain.

You agree to advocate on behalf of a patient with severe mental illness who has been excluded by his family.

A young woman presents to you with recurring abdominal pain. Physical examination and special investigations, including blood tests and ultrasound, are normal. You decide to discuss with her the possibility that there may be a psychological aspect to her problem.

2. **Communication skills:** Family doctors adopt person-centred approaches to assess, manage and support people with mental health problems.

Good communication skills are essential for effective consultations, for whatever conditions our patients present. They are of particular importance in the field of mental health, where patients are often in a state of vulnerability and uncertainty, and need the highest quality of care.

---

**Core competencies**

- Family doctors listen actively and are respectful and non-judgemental at all times.
- Family doctors use information-gathering skills to elicit symptoms as well as patients' ideas, concerns and expectations.
- Family doctors express empathy and compassion for their patients' distress.
- Family doctors manage problems and make culturally appropriate shared treatment plans with patients.
- Family doctors use effective information-giving skills in meeting their patients' needs.

---

**Example**

You ask your patient with abdominal pain what she thinks might be causing her pain and how much of a worry it is to her. You ask her what sort of help she is hoping you can give her. She tells you that she doesn't know what is causing the pain but it is very hard to bear. She is particularly worried because her mother had a pain like this last year and it turned out to be stomach cancer. She wants you to take the pain away and make sure she hasn't got cancer. You listen carefully to her story, and tell her that you can see how difficult this must be for her. You explain that the tests you have already done show that she does not have cancer, and that she is generally in good physical health. You tell her that, nevertheless, you know her pain is very real, and you will help her to manage it. Then you ask her about her home life. She bursts into tears. She tells you how much she misses her mother, and how difficult she is finding it to care for her three young children without her mother's help.

3. **Assessment:** Family doctors identify and diagnose common mental health problems, and can identify severe mental health problems and assess risk.

Once we have identified our core values, and developed our communication skills, we can then begin to assess or diagnose the various different mental health problems that our patients may present to us.

We know that patients present mental health problems in many different ways. They will often present with physical symptoms. In some cultures, emotional distress may be related to personal problems or shortcomings, while in other cultures patients may relate distress to their social or economic circumstances. Some may be concerned that unusual and distressing experiences are the result of religious persecution or spirit possession.

We are capable of considering probable causes and possible effects, including the risks they may pose to patients and to others.

---

**Core competencies**

- Family doctors are aware of different cultural presentations and understandings of mental health problems.
- Family doctors diagnose common mental health problems, including depressive disorders, anxiety disorders and substance misuse.
- Family doctors distinguish common mental disorders from normal responses to adverse and traumatic events, e.g. grief reactions.
- Family doctors assess how psychosocial stressors and supports affect the patient's mental health.
- Family doctors assess how mental health problems affect the patient's daily functioning.

---

- Family doctors undertake risk assessments, including suicide and self-harm, neglect, risk to others and risk from others.
- Family doctors are aware of severe mental health problems, including dementias, psychotic disorders and personality disorders.
- Family doctors understand interactions between physical and mental health, especially for patients with long-term conditions, multimorbidity or unexplained physical symptoms.
- Family doctors undertake physical health assessments and management of identified comorbid problems for patients with severe mental illness.

For family doctors who have additional training and experience in this field, here are the elements of advanced practice:

- Family doctors know the prevalence and risk factors for common mental disorders.
- Family doctors apply and interpret common mental health assessment questionnaires to assist in the diagnosis of common mental health problems.
- Family doctors diagnose dementias, psychotic disorders and personality disorders, usually with support from specialist mental health services.
- Family doctors assess a patient's mental capacity to make informed decisions about consenting and refusing types of medical care.

**Examples**

Continuing to care for the young woman with abdominal pain, you know that it is common for patients to present mental distress with physical symptoms, particularly if they think that family doctors are only interested in physical health. You are aware that anxiety and depressive disorders are relatively common amongst women caring for young children, but you also consider that this patient's main problem may be a grief reaction following her mother's death. You gently ask her whether she has thoughts of harming herself, and are assured that she would not do so because her children need her.

You next see an older man whose son is concerned that he is becoming increasingly forgetful. He has wandered out of the family home on several occasions and been unable to find his way back again. Twice he has started to cook something on the fire and then left it unattended. His son is worried he will burn the house down. You undertake a simple cognitive assessment with the aid of a validated questionnaire, which indicates that it is probably dementia. You arrange for a set of blood tests and refer him to specialist mental health services for further assessment.

Then you see a middle-aged man who has a longstanding diagnosis of schizophrenia. He asks you if the voices he sometimes hears are evil spirits, and you assure him they are not. You decide it is time to check his cardio-metabolic risk factors. You ask him about his smoking, alcohol, dietary and exercise habits and his current use of antipsychotic medication, measure his blood pressure, calculate his body-mass index, and arrange for blood tests to check his glucose and lipid levels.

> **4. Management:** Family doctors manage people with common mental health problems, and the physical health of people with severe mental health problems.

As family doctors, we have the ability to offer a wide range of psychosocial and pharmacological interventions to help our patients with mental health problems. At the simplest level, good communication skills, as set out in domain 2 above, will go a long way to alleviate our patients' suffering and distress. But there is a lot more that we can do to help patients manage their problems.

---

**Core competencies**

- Family doctors apply cognitive, behavioural and psychosocial interventions, e.g. psychoeducation, motivational interviewing, stress management, behavioural activation, problem solving and mindfulness.
- Family doctors explain and prescribe antidepressant and anxiolytic medication, consistent with evidence-based guidelines.
- Family doctors are aware of the uses of antipsychotic and antidementia medications and their principal side effects.
- Family doctors manage the physical health of people with severe mental illness, including infectious diseases, chronic respiratory diseases and cardio-metabolic interventions.
- Family doctors manage the mental health of people with chronic physical conditions.
- Family doctors engage and support families and carers of people with mental health problems.
- Family doctors ensure an appropriate plan for follow-up is in place.

---

For family doctors who have additional training and experience in this field, advanced practice may also include prescribing antipsychotic and antidementia medications, usually with support from specialist mental health services.

## Examples

The young woman with abdominal pain realises that grief for her mother is probably her main problem. You discuss treatment options with her, and it is clear that she would prefer non-drug approaches. You propose behavioural activation, and recommend an online meditation app. You help her to identify and involve supportive family and friends. You arrange to see her again next week.

Having assessed your patient with schizophrenia, you find that he is overweight, and has raised blood pressure. You give him information on healthy eating, and encourage him to take regular physical exercise. You advise him that he may need antihypertensive medication, being mindful of possible drug interactions with his antipsychotic medication.

An older woman with rheumatoid disease tells you that she is tired all the time and is finding no enjoyment in her life. She would prefer to be dead. You take a careful history, including assessment of risk, and diagnose severe depression. After discussing her problems with her and her daughter, you prescribe a course of antidepressant medication. You regularly monitor her suicide risk and response to medication, and consider referral to specialist mental health services if her symptoms do not improve.

5. **Collaboration and referral:** Family doctors use a range of available options and resources for the care of people with mental health problems, and tailor them to their patients' and carers' needs.

While there is a great deal we can do ourselves to help patients with mental health problems, it is also important for family doctors to be aware of who else can help, and to know how to make best use of other available resources. These include the patient themselves, their family and social networks, the wider primary care team, and mental health specialists.

---

### Core competencies

- Family doctors involve the patient as a resource for their own care.
- Family doctors involve the patient's family and social network as resources for patient care.

---

- Family doctors involve the wider primary care team, e.g. nurses, case managers and psychological therapists, as resources for patient care.
- Family doctors share the care of patients with severe or complex mental health problems with specialist mental health services.
- Family doctors initiate the management of emergency presentations in people with mental health problems.
- Family doctors are aware of mandatory legal requirements and know how to access legal interventions, for example, in cases of violence involving patients with mental health problems.

Family doctors may also involve community and voluntary agencies (including faith centres) and welfare agencies (such as social care, housing, education and the financial benefit system) as resources for patient care.

**Examples**

For your patient with schizophrenia, you involve his brother in plans for his new exercise routine. Together they decide to join a local walking group. You also ask his mental health specialist for advice on whether his current antipsychotic medication is affecting his weight gain.

When your older patient with rheumatoid disease is beginning to feel less depressed, you discuss with her how she has successfully tackled difficult problems in the past. You also ask your nurse to advise her on practical help in her home.

For the patient with severe mental illness who has been excluded by his family, with his consent you contact the leader of his local faith community, to discuss how to encourage the family to exercise their social obligations. You also ask the local police force to investigate allegations of violence towards this patient.

6. **Reflective practice:** Family doctors take care of their own health and well-being.

In order to give our patients the best possible care, we need to take good care of ourselves. An exhausted or stressed family doctor is going to be of much less benefit to their patients, and may even put them at risk.

---

**Core competencies**

- Family doctors know the limits of their own knowledge and skills.
- Family doctors actively seek support and advice if they are out of their depth, cognitively or emotionally.
- Family doctors nurture their own mental health.

---

**Examples**

A young man tells you that his neighbours are watching him all the time and strangers are following him when he walks down the street. You are unsure whether these are ideas of reference, related to severe anxiety, drug misuse or a possible psychotic illness. You decide to refer him urgently for a specialist mental health opinion.

You are distressed after a patient tells you that she was abused by her father as a child and is now in a relationship with a man who is frequently violent towards her. You arrange to meet with one of your colleagues after work, to talk about how you are feeling.

You expect yourself to be a 'good enough' doctor, and do not strive to be perfect. You maintain a balance between your work and your home life, spending time with your loved ones. You find time for meditation or prayer. You make sure you have regular enjoyable activities in your life, such as reading, exercise and socialising.

# Implications for service delivery

Now that you have read these competencies, across the six domains of practice, it is worth pausing to reflect on them for a few moments.

The first question to ask yourself is: 'How much of this am I already capable of?' We are confident that everyone reading this chapter will find several areas in which they feel competent. We hope that many of you will consider yourself competent in most of them.

For those competencies or standards where you find you are less confident, there are two further questions to ask. The first is: 'Is this something I can address myself, with some further education or training?' If so, at the end of this chapter we indicate a set of resources to help you to gain further knowledge and experience. This is also a question for educators, considering what subjects to cover in training programmes for family medicine residents, or when setting up continuing professional development courses for established family doctors.

For some family doctors, particularly those working in low and middle income countries, it may be that the circumstances in which you are working make it difficult to put even the highest level of knowledge and skills into practice. So a further question is: 'What help do I need to be able to provide good mental health care for my patients?' You may decide that you need better premises, with more space and opportunity for confidential discussions; or more health care workers, to allow you to spend more time with each patient; or better access to specialist mental health services. For these types of solutions you may well need the help of policy makers to develop local, regional or national initiatives to integrate mental health and primary care.

We are aware that in some regions, for example in Central Asia, the diagnosis and management of common mental disorders are not yet considered part of the family doctor's role. However, we are confident that they should be. We encourage and support family doctors across the world to work with professional colleagues in related disciplines, and with regional and national policy makers, to make sure that these core competencies are implemented into their routine clinical practice. As examples, we recommend:

- the WHO-led initiative to integrate mental health into primary health care across the Eastern Mediterranean region;
- the collaboration between primary care clinicians and the Pan-American Health Organization (PAHO) to provide a series of mhGAP training programmes for family doctors across Brazil;
- the collaboration between psychiatrists and family doctors from Australia and China to deliver a mental health training programme for GPs in Guangzhou province, China.

We also expect that these competencies will be useful for those wishing to engage with audit and research in primary mental health care. Examples include: audits of current practice regarding mental health diagnoses and the range of existing treatment options; research into cultural variations of the presentation of mental health problems in primary care settings; research into the clinical effectiveness of non-drug interventions for depression; and research into the cost-effectiveness of family doctor-led physical health care for patients living with psychosis.

The WONCA Working Party for Mental Health will be pleased to support family doctors, educators, policy makers, and researchers seeking to develop initiatives to improve core competencies. We have experience of doing so in different regions across the world including Eastern Europe, Latin America and Asia-Pacific.

# Educational material

### Case study

This case study is one we have discussed earlier in this chapter. We review it here, to give you an opportunity to check your own knowledge and understanding. Please consider your responses to the questions we pose, before turning to the answers we give.

A young woman presents to you with recurring abdominal pain. Physical examination and special investigations, including blood tests and ultrasound, are normal.

*What should you do next?*

- Reassure her that everything is normal and tell her there is no need to see you again unless her pain gets worse? OR
- Discuss with her the possibility that there may be a psychological aspect to her problem?

Reassurance is unlikely to be helpful; the patient may well think that you are not taking her or her problems seriously. It is more useful to explore her problems in greater detail.

Using the standard consultation technique of ICE (ideas, concerns and expectations) you ask your patient with abdominal pain what she thinks might be causing her pain and how much of a worry it is to her. You ask her what sort of help she is hoping you can give her.

She tells you that she doesn't know what is causing the pain but it is very hard to bear. She is particularly worried because her mother had a pain like this last year and it turned out to be stomach cancer. She wants you to take the pain away and make sure she hasn't got cancer.

You listen carefully to her story, and tell her that you can see how difficult this must be for her. You explain that the tests you have already done show that she does not have cancer, and that she is generally in good physical health. You tell her that, nevertheless, you know her pain is very real, and you will help her to manage it. Then you ask her about her home life.

She bursts into tears. She tells you how much she misses her mother, and how difficult she is finding it to care for her three young children without her mother's help.

*What is the likely diagnosis?*
- Grief reaction? OR
- Anxiety disorder?

You know that it is common for patients to present mental distress with physical symptoms, particularly if they think that family doctors are only interested in physical health. You are aware that anxiety and depressive disorders are relatively common amongst women caring for young children, but you also consider that this patient's main problem may be a grief reaction following her mother's death. You gently ask her whether she has thoughts of harming herself, and are assured that she would not do so because her children need her.

She realises that grief for her mother is probably her main problem.

*What is your best management plan?*
- Prescribe an antidepressant? OR
- Discuss the patient's preferred treatment options?

Antidepressant medication could be helpful for your patient, although it would not be the first-line treatment for an uncomplicated grief reaction. We consider this further in the next chapter.

It is valuable to give your patient as much choice as possible, as this will enhance her sense of capacity. You discuss treatment options with her, and it is clear that she would prefer non-drug approaches. You propose behavioural activation, and recommend an online meditation app. You help her to identify and involve supportive family and friends. You arrange to see her again next week.

## Multiple choice questions

For family doctors caring for patients with mental health problems:

1. Which one of the following is evidence of competent values?

   a. Family doctors consider physical health more important than mental health.

   b. Family doctors treat patients with mental health problems with dignity and respect.

    c.    Family doctors believe mental health problems are the patient's own fault.

    d.    Family doctors refer all patients with mental health problems to specialists.

2.    Which one of the following is *not* evidence of competent communication?

    a.    Family doctors listen actively and are respectful and non-judgemental at all times.

    b.    Family doctors use information-gathering skills to elicit symptoms as well as patients' ideas, concerns and expectations.

    c.    Family doctors express empathy and compassion for their patients' distress.

    d.    Family doctors tell patients how to manage their problems.

3.    Which one of the following is evidence of a competent assessment?

    a.    Family doctors ignore patients' cultural presentations and understandings of mental health problems.

    b.    Family doctors diagnose common mental health problems, including depressive disorders, anxiety disorders and substance misuse.

    c.    Family doctors make no distinctions between mental disorders and normal responses to adverse and traumatic events.

    d.    Family doctors ask specialists to undertake all risk assessments, including suicide and self-harm, neglect, risk to others and risk from others.

4.    Which one of the following is *not* evidence of competent management?

    a.    Family doctors ask psychologists to undertake all cognitive, behavioural and psychosocial interventions.

    b.    Family doctors explain and prescribe antidepressant and anxiolytic medication, consistent with evidence-based guidelines.

    c.    Family doctors manage the physical health of people with severe mental illness.

    d.    Family doctors manage the mental health of people with chronic physical conditions.

5.  Which one of the following is *not* evidence of competent reflective practice?

    a.  Family doctors know the limits of their own knowledge and skills.
    b.  Family doctors actively seek support and advice if they are out of their depth.
    c.  Family doctors use alcohol as a safety valve when they feel stressed.
    d.  Family doctors nurture their own mental health.

You will find the answers to these MCQs on page 171.

# Further reading and e-resources

The chapters which follow will give you plenty of material, to help you build your knowledge and skills in caring for primary care patients with mental health problems. Here are some additional resources that you may also find helpful.

## General

- Gold B, Green L (eds). Integrating Behavioral Health in Primary Care. Springer. 2019.
- WHO mhGAP Intervention Guide 2.0. www.who.int/mental_health/mhgap/mhGAP_intervention_guide_02/en/
- WONCA-WHO. Integrating Mental Health in Primary Care. 2008. www.who.int/mental_health/policy/Mental%20health%20+%20primary%20care-%20final%20low-res%20120109.pdf

## Values

- Prince M, Patel V, Saxena S, et al. No health without mental health. *Lancet* 2007, 370: 859–77.
- WHO Quality Rights Toolkit. 2012. www.who.int/mental_health/publications/QualityRights_toolkit/en/
- World Federation for Mental Health. Report on Dignity in Mental Health. 2015. www.rcpsych.ac.uk/pdf/WMHD_report_2015_vertical_v7.pdf
- World Psychiatric Association Bill of Rights for Persons with Mental Illness. 2017. http://wpanet.org/WMMD16/BillofRights_MentalIllness_FINAL.pdf

## Communication skills

- Coll X, Papageorgiou A, Stanley A, Tarbuck A. (eds) Communication Skills in Mental Health Care. Radcliffe. 2012.
- Silverman J, Kurtz S, Draper J. Skills for Communicating with Patients. 3rd edition. Radcliffe Medical Press. 2013.

## Assessment

- Chitnis A, Dowrick C, Byng R et al. Guidance for health professionals on medically unexplained symptoms. Royal College of General Practitioners and Royal College of Psychiatrists. 2014.
- French P, Shiers D, Jones P. GP Guidance: Early detection of emerging psychosis. RCGP/RCPsych. 2014.

## Management

- Asen E, Tomson D, Young V, Tomson P. Ten Minutes for the Family: Systemic Interventions for Primary Care. Routledge. 2004.
- David L. Using CBT in General Practice: the 10 Minute CBT Handbook. 2nd edition. Scion. 2013.
- Improving the Physical Health of Adults with Severe Mental Illness: Essential Actions (OP100). Royal College of Psychiatrists. 2016.
- Robinson P, Gould D, Strosahl K. Real Behaviour Change in Primary Care: Improving Patient Outcomes and Increasing Job Satisfaction. New Harbinger Publications. 2011.
- Stuart M, Lieberman J. The Fifteen Minute Hour: Therapeutic Talk in Primary Care. 5th edition. Radcliffe. 2015.
- WHO guidelines: Management of physical health conditions in adults with severe mental disorder. www.who.int/mental_health/evidence/guidelines_severe_mental_disorders_web_note_2018/en/

## Collaboration and referral

- Cochrane Collaboration. Collaborative care for people with depression and anxiety. 2012. www.cochrane.org/CD006525/DEPRESSN_collaborative-care-for-people-with-depression-and-anxiety
- RCGP Collaborative Care and Support Planning Toolkit. www.rcgp.org.uk/clinical-and-research/toolkits/collaborative-care-and-support-planning-toolkit.aspx
- WHO. Scalable psychological interventions for people in communities affected by adversity. 2017. http://apps.who.int/iris/bitstream/10665/254581/1/WHO-MSD-MER-17.1-eng.pdf

## Reflective practice

- Dowrick C. Wellbeing blog: www.wellbecoming.blogspot.com
- Epstein R. Attending: Medicine, Mindfulness and Humanity. Simon & Schuster. 2017.
- Foundation for Positive Mental Health. www.foundationforpositivemental health.com
- Rowe L, Kidd M. First Do No Harm: Being a Resilient Doctor in the 21st Century. McGraw-Hill Medical. 2009.

## Competency documents

Our guidance is consistent with mental health-related competency work undertaken elsewhere, including:

- Brazilian Society for Family and Community Medicine. *Curriculo Baseado em Competências para Medicina de Família e Communidade.* 2015.
- European Union of General Practitioners (UEMO): www.uemo.eu/mission/
- Miller B, Gilchrist E, Ross K, et al. Core Competencies for Behavioral Health Providers Working in Primary Care. Colorado Consensus Conference. 2016.
- Royal College of General Practitioners. Curriculum: Professional and Clinical Modules. Section 3.10 Care of people with mental health problems. 2016. www.rcgp.org.uk/training-exams/gp-curriculum-overview/online-curriculum/managing-complex-care/3-10-mental-health-problems.aspx
- University College London competence frameworks for the delivery of effective psychological interventions: www.ucl.ac.uk/pals/research/cehp/research-groups/core/competence-frameworks
- WHO mhGAP training manuals. 2017. www.who.int/mental_health/mhgap/training_manuals/en/

# Advice and support

If you would like further advice or support to put these competencies in practice, please contact WONCA Mental Health Consultancies on mhconsult@wonca.net.

# Chapter 2

# DEPRESSION

An evidence-based first
consultation

**Bruce Arroll, Weng Yee Chin, Fiona
Moir, Vicki Mount and Christopher
Dowrick**

# Key points

1. Depression is common in primary care.
2. Most patients with depression present with somatic symptoms.
3. Open the consultation by asking about mental health alongside physical health.
4. Avoid diagnostic labels at the first visit.
5. Understand why many doctors don't make a mental health diagnosis.
6. Reflect on the difference between being given a diagnosis, versus just being heard and understood.
7. Use two questions as a quick way to rule out depression.
8. Explore further if there is a positive response to either of the depression questions.
9. Remember that high depression inventory scores do not necessarily signify depression.
10. Use empathic listening and consider non-drug therapies first.
11. Consider if antidepressants should be prescribed on the first visit.
12. Be aware that early prescription of antidepressants might risk "medicalising" the patient's suffering.
13. Organise a phone call to the patient between visits.
14. Arrange early follow-up, ideally one week later.

### 1. Depression is common in primary care.

Depression is commonly understood as a psychological condition characterised by at least two weeks of low mood that is present across most situations. It is often accompanied by low self-esteem, loss of interest in normally enjoyable activities, low energy, and pain without a clear cause.

The 14-country World Health Organisation Collaborative Study on Psychological Problems in General Health Care (WHO PPGHC) estimated that about 14% (range 2.6%–15.9%) of individuals in primary health care centres suffered from major depression.[1] The Longitudinal Investigation of Depressive Outcomes (LIDO) in Primary Care study reported a similar prevalence for depression in primary care of 13% (range 4%–23%).[2]

### 2. Most patients with depression present with somatic symptoms.

Of patients with depression, 45% to 95% present with somatic symptoms and 11% do not report any psychological symptoms.[3]

It may be easier to screen for the somatic symptoms of depression such as changes in sleep, energy, appetite and movement. There may also be an increase or decrease in the amount of speech, and perhaps changes in levels of concentration. This can be followed by asking about changes in mood and pleasure, along with guilty and suicidal feelings.[4]

If the patient identifies a change in their mood, you can ask if they have been under any stress lately, as people experiencing stress often answer "yes" to a question about mood. Filling out a depression inventory instrument can be very useful, and many of these are easy to use in a primary care setting (e.g. Patient Health Questionnaire [PHQ-9], Hospital Anxiety and Depression Scale – Depression [HAD-D], Beck Depression Inventory [BDI]).[5] Patients may be more accepting of a mood or distress diagnosis if they have filled out a form themselves.

### 3. Open the consultation by asking about mental health along-side physical health.

Given that most consultations start with a physical presentation, clinicians need to raise the possibility of psychological as well as physical causes, especially when the symptoms do not clearly lead to a physical diagnosis. Symptoms such as insomnia, fatigue and irritability require further exploration of mood and the quickest way to do this is by using a mood inventory.[6]

This can be done directly by asking: "How has your mood or your spirits been lately?" Alternatively, it can be done more indirectly, by first asking about sleep, energy, concentration and enjoyment of life, and depending on the answers, then going on to ask directly about depression. A further useful technique here can be to normalise: "Often when people have been experiencing a reduction in their sleep and concentration, they also notice they've been feeling a bit down – have you noticed any changes in your mood recently?" This is not screening, but case finding, as the patient's symptoms indicate that there could be a mood component. Screening asymptomatic patients for depression is controversial and not recommended.[7]

If unsure, then you can ask the patient to fill out a depression inventory (e.g. PHQ-9). If the score is low, pursue the physical health aspects. If higher, you can broach the subject by saying: "This questionnaire suggests you may be having problems with your mood – what do you think?" Many patients will be quite open to the doctor exploring their psychological concerns further. However, some patients can be somatically oriented rather than psychologically oriented, and unlikely to accept a mental health diagnosis. It is important not to become adversarial at this point;

simply raising the possibility of a mental health component may be sufficient to allow the patient to discuss psychological matters later.

### 4. Avoid diagnostic labels at the first visit.

Making a mental health diagnosis in the primary care setting can be challenging. As summed up by one GP: "we actually risk-manage and live in this glorious twilight zone of uncertainty."[8] A diagnosis of depression may be more safely made over more than one visit.[9] This is a common primary care strategy and is known as using time as the diagnostic test.[10] In practical terms, if the patient is not making rapid progress emotionally then they are likely to have a mood disorder rather than a short lived emotional crisis.

Applying the label of depression at the first consultation can be problematic as it can be upsetting news to receive, and giving a label such as depression as part of an initial brief primary care consultation is likely to be wrong. This may be one of the worst days in the patient's life and partial or complete resolution may occur with time.[11]

A key challenge encountered is in case definition and deciding where the cut-off lies between psychological distress and clinical depression. Primary care doctors are usually able to recognise patients experiencing distress as a result of problems in their lives, but find it more difficult to decide whether the issues are clinically significant and whether or not to make an explicit mental health diagnosis.[9] A meta-analysis by Mitchell et al. found that while primary care doctors are good at ruling out depression (specificity of 81%), we are 50% more likely to make an incorrect diagnosis of depression (a false positive) than to diagnose depression correctly (a true positive).[12]

The issue of distress is acknowledged in primary care but there has been limited work on how to measure it. A questionnaire from the Netherlands, the 4-DSQ, has been validated and measures distress, anxiety, depression and somatisation.[13,14] The main limitation is that it has 50 questions, making it less useful in regular short primary care consultations.

### 5. Understand why many doctors don't make a mental health diagnosis.

There are several reasons why doctors may not make a mental health diagnosis even if they are aware that the patient is experiencing psychological distress.

Doctors are usually trained to explore the physical aspects first based on the premise that it is bad practice to miss a physical diagnosis but less problematic to miss a mental health diagnosis.[8] In addition, general practitioners tend to think in terms of problems rather than diagnoses, and may not label a patient with depression unless they plan to treat it.[15,16] We feel there is merit in this approach of describing the specific functional problem, e.g. "distress with reduced motivation", or "excess time in bed and excessive use of substances". It then becomes clear what issues need attention.

In some countries, general practitioners are not allowed to make a mental health diagnosis, and are expected to refer all suspected cases to a psychiatrist. In these situations, we suggest advising simple behavioural activation which may help the patient to manage their symptoms, while waiting to see the psychiatrist.

Some doctors don't like managing mental health issues.[8] Some are reluctant to explore psychosocial issues in case they open up Pandora's Box.[8] Ironically at the bottom of Pandora's Box lies hope. Some avoid doing so due to a lack of confidence or feeling under skilled in raising mental health issues.[17] There may be issues related to the clinician's own emotional state or their workload – as described in a poem by GP poet Glenn Colquhoun, "I saw a young woman for a repeat prescription. Her story was so large I knew not to ask about it in the morning when the day is fragile with need."[18] Here the clinician is not feeling emotionally or practically able to deal with the anticipated complex issues being presented by a distressed patient.[19]

Other doctors have concerns about stigma for the patient[8] whilst others are concerned about the impact on future insurance claims if a diagnosis of depression is recorded in the medical records. In addition, some doctors may take the view that many conditions currently diagnosed as major depressive disorder, especially those related to other forms of loss, are better understood within a model of grief that does not require drug treatment.[20,21]

### 6. Reflect on the difference between being given a diagnosis, versus just being heard and understood.

There is considerable overlap in symptoms between depression and anxiety. The MaGPie study from New Zealand found 18.1% of primary care patients met the criteria for depression over the past 12 months but 56% of them had a co-existing DSM IV level anxiety and 20% a substance use and dependence disorder.[22] Some people with medically unexplained symptoms may be anxious or depressed. There may be a new term in the ICD-11 called "anxious depression" which includes mixed anxiety and depression.[23]

Developing a shared and respectful understanding of the patient's problems, including relevant cultural aspects, is important. This involves establishing rapport, obtaining the patient's trust, enabling patients to tell their stories and allowing a healing partnership to form.[24] There are structured approaches to enhancing the clinician's communication skills, such as asking five questions (BATHE approach): "What is going on in your life?"; "How do you feel about that?"; "What troubles you most about this?"; "How are you handling that?"; "That must be difficult for you".[24] Such frameworks can be extremely useful, but it is necessary to note the importance of incorporating them in a genuine, rather than a formulaic, manner.

Active listening is recommended.[25] The late Professor Ian McWhinney said, "the greatest single problem in clinical interviewing is the failure to let the patient tell their story."[26] The patient's context is also important and in addition to the mental health concerns, consideration of loneliness, co-morbid physical conditions, family violence, sexual and physical abuse, crime, war, migration and homelessness may be needed. Strosahl makes the point that life constriction precedes or accompanies mental health issues. It is important to find out what is happening with the patient's work, friends, partner(s) and family as well as recreation. This is captured in the contextual interview known as the work/love/play questionnaire.[27]

### 7. Use two questions as a quick way to rule out depression.

This is different from general screening, as our recommendation is to use these questions for the patient with somatic presenting symptoms for which the physical diagnosis is elusive. The more physical symptoms there are, the greater the likelihood of a mental health component. The prevalence of depression in such a clinical setting will be higher than in an asymptomatic screening population and the activity is thus considered to be "case finding".[28]

The two questions are:

1. Have you felt depressed down or hopeless for all or most of the past month?
2. Have you lost interest or pleasure in all or most activities over the past month?

A negative score for both questions almost always rules out depression.[29]

**8. Explore further if there is a positive response to either of the depression questions.**

If patients answer "yes" to either question, they may be depressed. A PHQ-9 or other depression inventory will assist in giving a measure of severity.[30] General practitioners should always consider suicide risk and the patient's functional ability. The PHQ-9 has questions on both suicide and functioning. Among those in the general population who commit suicide, up to 83% may have had contact with general practitioners in the year prior to death and up to 20% may commit suicide within one day of seeing their GP. The corresponding figures are 41% and 9% for psychiatric inpatient care. Among those who die by suicide, contact with health services is common before death.[31] The National Institute for Health and Care Excellence (NICE) (UK guidelines group) recommends, "Always ask people with depression directly about suicidal ideation and intent if there is a risk of self-harm or suicide."[32]

An informal assessment of function can be made by asking the patient about difficulties experienced in social, occupational and family situations.

At this point it is important to check for any past history of mania as about 10% of the primary care population prescribed antidepressant medication actually have undetected bipolar disorder.[33] Assessment is also recommended for alcohol and drug use.

**9. Remember that high depression inventory scores do not necessarily signify depression.**

The PHQ-9 indicates levels of distress, and patients can have very high scores and not be depressed.[34] Research undertaken in the UK suggests that a score of 12 or more on the PHQ-9 (the maximum score is 27) may be a better cut-off to use when deciding whether or not to offer active treatment (usually non-drug first). This score demonstrated greater specificity, and the same sensitivity as a score of 10 for major depression in a UK population.[35]

There is evidence that 60% of primary care patents will have a resolution of their depressive symptoms over one year even if the depressive symptoms are not recognised at the first visit.[36] Many patients' scores are already lower in the following week, due either to regression to the mean or to having discussed their symptoms with a clinician (Dr Michael Balint called this "the doctor as the drug").[37]

### 10. Use empathic listening and consider non-drug therapies first.

We encourage you to begin with non-drug therapies for most patients. NICE guidelines recommend not starting medication at lower levels of severity of depression, but to use non-drug therapies.[38]

Consider trying low intensity psychosocial interventions first. These may include:

1. sleep hygiene;
2. individualised self-help principles of CBT;
3. computerised CBT with a facilitator;
4. problem solving therapy;
5. behavioural activation, examples are seeing people they have avoided contacting, doing social activities and increasing their level of exercise;
6. physical activity (recommended in groups);
7. mindfulness;
8. psychoeducation – explaining the causes of depression can normalise the diagnosis and reduce self-stigma and reduce blame;[39]
9. group therapy has been shown to be effective in developing countries.[40]

We discuss non-drug interventions in more detail in Chapter 3.

A Cochrane review found that exercise is moderately more effective than a control intervention for reducing symptoms of depression, but no more effective than psychological or pharmacological treatments.[41] In a 2016 randomised controlled trial (RCT), Hallgren found that exercise is beneficial for depression even when it is light (yoga and stretching) as opposed to moderate and vigorous and when conducted once per week.[42] Furthermore, there can be cardiovascular and metabolic benefits for patients with depression.

Acceptance and commitment therapy (ACT) is a third wave cognitive behavioural therapy that includes a mindfulness component. It uses a transdiagnostic approach and patients are considered to be "stuck" rather than depressed or anxious.[43] Limited time is spent on diagnosis when used in primary care (where it is known as "FACT" – focussed acceptance and commitment therapy), with the emphasis being on using that time for therapy, as it is known that many patients do not return for a second visit.[27]

### 11. Consider if antidepressants should be prescribed on the first visit.

There is currently an absence of evidence on what treatment to start at the first visit. It appears likely that the magnitude of benefit of antidepressant medication increases with the severity of depression symptoms and may be minimal or non-existent, on average, in patients with mild or moderate symptoms. For patients with very severe depression, the benefit of medications over placebo appears to be more substantial.[44-46]As most patients in primary care are in the mild to moderate range and many of those in the severe range will become mild to moderate fairly quickly, most patients are less likely to benefit from antidepressants. Patients may be more likely to benefit from antidepressant medication if they have symptoms of anxiety as well as depression.[47]

### 12. Be aware that early prescription of antidepressants might risk "medicalising" the patient's suffering.

There are many risks of early prescribing: many patients will get adverse effects; the patient may not come back; they may have difficulty in stopping their medication or they may take an overdose.[46]

Therefore we do not suggest using antidepressants routinely to treat persistent sub-threshold depressive symptoms or mild depression because the risk-benefit ratio is poor. Most people do not benefit from antidepressants, and improvements are more likely to be a placebo response rather than a medication response. For mild to moderate depressive symptoms, the placebo response will be about eight times more likely than a true drug response.[44] As most patients are likely to get a placebo response, they are likely to give the medication the credit rather than their changed world view or increase in exercise and/or social activities. They may expect medications the next time they feel distressed, thereby medicalising their suffering.[48]

Problems associated with withdrawal symptoms when trying to stop these medications also need to be considered as it can lead to the unnecessary long term use of antidepressants.[46] NICE advises avoiding drug treatment unless there is a past history of moderate or severe depression that persists after other interventions, or sub-threshold symptoms that have been present for a long period, typically at least two years.[38]

### 13. Organise a phone call to the patient between visits.

In a randomised controlled trial, nurse-led telehealth care was shown to improve clinical outcomes and patient satisfaction,[49] therefore we recommend a follow-up phone call as part of routine practice. In each telephone call the clinic's nurse asked the patient about any concerns regarding the antidepressant medication, offered suggestions on how to deal with minor side effects, and emphasised the importance of taking the medication regularly. The nurse offered emotional support and helped patients identify activities that they were willing to try to be more active and to find pleasure. Furthermore, it was reported that the nurse could also address issues about other medical conditions and discuss the patient's overall health.[49] In some health services a nurse may not be available. A study in Germany used Health Care Assistants for this task.[50]

### 14. Arrange early follow-up, ideally one week later.

There is no evidence base for choosing such a time interval but we are influenced by the comments of a UK GP in the "An insider's guide to depression" where she says, "see us frequently at first, a week is a long time in a Dali landscape. Three weeks are almost unimaginable."[51]

We acknowledge that weekly follow-up may not be within the resources of some health services and that factors such as severity may influence the discussion.

## Disclaimer

The authors all work in high income countries and are aware that some of our suggestions may be not be feasible in all countries. Issues of language, war, migration, distance, cultures that prefer verbal rather than written transactions, staffing, translation of questionnaires and limited roles for primary care practitioners in mental health will all modify the ability of some practitioners to follow our suggestions.

## Educational material

### Case study
A 48-year-old woman, Mrs A, presents to you with insomnia and fatigue. She has previously slept well, but over the past few months has been waking early in the morning and is unable to return to sleep. The resulting fatigue is affecting her work as a typist at the local police department.

There are no significant findings on physical examination or investigations, including blood tests.

*What should you do next?*
1.  Reassure her that there is no sinister cause for her symptoms, and prescribe sleeping tablets to mitigate the symptoms.
2.  Ask two questions to check for depression.

Prescribing sleeping tablets at this stage may offer temporary respite but is unlikely to address the underlying issue. It is more useful to explore psychosocial causes for her symptoms.

You explore Mrs A's symptoms further using the consultation technique of ICE (ideas, concerns and expectations) to ask what she thinks might be causing her sleeplessness.

She tells you she has been under extra stress at work lately, after some colleagues left the department and were not replaced. This makes her feel undervalued. She wakes in the early hours of the morning thinking about work and is unable to return to sleep.

You ask the two questions about depression:

"Have you felt depressed, down or hopeless for all or most of the past month?"

"Have you lost interest or pleasure in all or most activities over the past month?"

Mrs A answers "yes" to both questions, suggesting she has a mood issue. To determine the magnitude, you ask her to complete a PHQ-9. She scores 16, indicating a moderate to severe mood problem. Importantly, she denies any thoughts of self-harm.

*How do you communicate these results to Mrs A?*
1.  Tell her she meets the criteria for depression.
2.  Suggest that she is distressed and "stuck".

Remember, a high depression inventory score at the first visit may signify distress rather than depression. Many patients will have a lower score if the questionnaire is repeated the following week. Labelling a patient with depression at this stage may be premature.

You explain to Mrs A that her score indicates she is suffering significant distress. Using the technique of empathic listening, you ask her how she is coping with the symptoms.

She tells you she is drinking a bottle of wine every night to help her sleep. She has stopped exercising and seeing her friends due to the fatigue.

She agrees that these strategies are not helpful and acknowledges they may be making it worse. She asks what treatment you would suggest.

*What treatment should you offer Mrs A?*
1. Low intensity psychosocial interventions.
2. Start an antidepressant.

Mrs A has not previously suffered from depression and it is reasonable to consider non-drug interventions first, with close follow-up. The likelihood of a benefit from antidepressant therapy reduces with decreasing symptom severity; mild depression is less likely to respond to pharmacotherapy alone. Although Mrs A has a moderate to severe score on the PHQ-9 today, it is reasonable to expect her score will improve in a short time with non-drug treatment. This option also reduces the risk of medicalising the patients' suffering and setting an expectation of a drug treatment for subsequent episodes of distress.

You ask Mrs A what she likes to do for exercise and she tells you she enjoys walking in the local park with her friend. Together, you agree that over the next week she will take three 30-minute walks. You ask her to rate the likelihood of doing this on a scale of 0–10 (0: not at all likely; 10: certain) and she rates it a 7, which you reflect back to motivate her further. She also agrees to have three alcohol-free days, and to try and reduce her wine intake on the other days.

*What follow-up should you offer Mrs A?*
1. Phone call follow-up with your nurse in three days, plus a review with you in one week.
2. Review in two weeks in your office.

Nurse-led telephone follow-up has been shown to improve clinical outcome and patient satisfaction. The nurse can offer emotional support to the patient along with an opportunity to discuss any other issues that may arise.

With Mrs A's consent, you introduce her to your nurse (a warm handover), and they agree your nurse will phone Mrs A in three days' time. Your nurse reports after this phone call that Mrs A is doing well and has managed one walk with her friend.

Mrs A returns to see you a week later. She tells you she enjoyed the walks and was pleased to have an opportunity to talk with her friend. Her sleep is still disrupted on some nights but she has been able to sleep until morning on two occasions. She feels better drinking less alcohol. You repeat her PHQ-9 inventory and she now has a score of 9.

You congratulate Mrs A on her progress and agree a follow-up plan for a nurse phone call in two weeks. You offer a planned review but Mrs A declines and will make an appointment if she feels it is necessary.

## Multiple choice questions

1. Which of the following patients is most likely to answer "yes" when asked the two questions to check for depression?

   a. A 36-year-old man with recent weight gain following an ankle fracture.
   b. A 48-year-old woman with a six-month history of abdominal pain, headache and fatigue with no localising signs on clinical examination and normal investigations.
   c. A 65-year-old man with new diarrhoea and weight loss over the past eight weeks.
   d. A 20-year-old woman with a new diagnosis of gonorrhoea.

2. When should you consider using the label "distressed" or "stuck" instead of diagnosing depression?

   a. After six months of antidepressant therapy in a patient with a first episode of depressive symptoms.
   b. If symptoms of depression persist after a two-week trial of low intensity psychosocial interventions.
   c. At the first presentation of mood symptoms suggestive of depression in a patient with no previous history of depression.
   d. At the first visit for a patient with low mood who has previously suffered a depressive episode.

3. Which of the following psychosocial interventions is most likely to improve mood symptoms in a patient who is "stuck"?

   a. Mindfulness for 20 minutes every day.
   b. Thirty minutes of moderate intensity exercise at least three times per week.
   c. Meeting a friend (also known as behavioural activation).

    d. Any of the above if the patient enjoys it and can commit to doing it regularly over the next week.

4. What is the best time frame and method for follow-up of a first presentation of mood symptoms of moderate severity?

    a. Phone review with the nurse in three to four days then follow-up appointment with the doctor in one week.

    b. Phone call from the doctor in one week.

    c. Appointment with the doctor in one week.

    d. Any of the above providing follow-up occurs within the first week of presentation.

5. What are the potential benefits of avoiding a label of depression at the first presentation?

    a. Avoid medicalising a normal distress reaction.

    b. Less likely to prescribe antidepressants and thus create an expectation of drug treatment for future episodes of distress.

    c. More likely to try psychosocial interventions.

    d. All of the above.

You will find the answers to these MCQs on page 171.

# References

1. Ormel J, Vonkorff M, Ustun B, et al. Common mental disorders and disability across cultures. *JAMA* 1994, 272:1741–1748.
2. Herrman H, Patrick DL, Diehr P, et al. Longitudinal investigation of depression outcomes in primary care in six countries: the LIDO study. Functional status, health service use and treatment of people with depressive symptoms. *Psychol Med* 2002, 32(5):889–902.
3. Simon GE, VonKorff M, Piccinelli M, et al. An international study of the relation between somatic symptoms and depression. *N Engl J Med* 1999, 341(18):1329–1335. doi: 10.1056/NEJM199910283411801.
4. Schumann I, Schneider A, Kantert C, et al. Physicians' attitudes, diagnostic process and barriers regarding depression diagnosis in primary care: a systematic review of qualitative studies. *Fam Pract* 2012, 29(3):255–263. doi: 10.1093/fampra/cmr092.
5. Mulrow CD, Williams JW, Jr., Gerety MB, et al. Case-finding instruments for depression in primary care settings. *Ann Intern Med* 1995, 122(12):913–921.
6. Kendrick A, Gunn J, Tylee A. Chapter 7 Depression in *Primary care mental health*, edited by L Gask, T Kendrick, R Peveler, CA Chew-Graham, Cambridge University Press, University Printing House, Cambridge, 87–102, 2018.

7.  Gilbody S, House AO, Sheldon TA. Screening and case finding instruments for depression [Systematic Review]. *Cochrane Database Syst Rev* 2005, (4): CD002792.
8.  Dew K, Dowell A, McLeod D, et al. "This glorious twilight zone of uncertainty": mental health consultations in general practice in New Zealand. *Soc Sci Med* 2005, 61(6):1189–1200. doi: 10.1016/j.socscimed.2005.01.025.
9.  Bushnell J. Frequency of consultations and general practitioner recognition of psychological symptoms. *Br J Gen Pract* 2004, 54(508):838–842.
10. Heneghan C, Glasziou P, Thompson M, et al. Diagnosis in general practice. Diagnostic strategies used in primary care. *BMJ* 2009, 338:1003–1006.
11. Frances A. Allen Frances at preventing over-diagnosis – what opened your eyes. *BMJ* podcast August 31 2018 https://itunes.apple.com/nz/podcast/the-bmj-podcast/id283916558?mt=2&i=1000418438338, 2018.
12. Mitchell AJ, Vaze A, Rao S. Clinical diagnosis of depression in primary care: a meta-analysis. *The Lancet* 2009, 374(9690):609–619.
13. Terluin B, Smits N, Miedema B. The English version of the four-dimensional symptom questionnaire (4DSQ) measures the same as the original Dutch questionnaire: a validation study. *Eur J Gen Pract* 2014, 20(4):320–326. doi: 10.3109/13814788.2014.905826.
14. Geraghty AW, Stuart B, Terluin B, et al. Distinguishing between emotional distress and psychiatric disorder in primary care attenders: a cross sectional study of the four-dimensional symptom questionnaire (4DSQ). *J Affect Disorders* 2015, 184:198–204.
15. Goldman LS, Nielsen NH, Champion HC, et al. Awareness, diagnosis, and treatment of depression. *J Gen Intern Med* 1999, 14(9):569–580. doi: 10.1046/j.1525-1497.1999.03478.x.
16. Rost K, Smith R, Matthews DB, et al. The deliberate misdiagnosis of major depression in primary care. *Arch Fam Med* 1994, 3(4):333–337. [published Online First: 1994/04/01].
17. Maxwell M, Harris F, Hibberd C, et al. A qualitative study of primary care professionals' views of case finding for depression in patients with diabetes or coronary heart disease in the UK. *BMC Fam Pract* 2013, 14:46. doi: 10.1186/1471-2296-14-46.
18. Colquhoun G. *Late love: sometimes doctors need saving as much as their patients.* Wellington, NZ: Bridget Williams Books, 2016.
19. Wilson H, Cunningham W. *Being a doctor: understanding medical practice.* London: Royal College of General Practitioners, 2014.
20. Parker G. Opening Pandora's box: how DSM-5 is coming to grief. *Acta Psychiatrica Scandinavica* 2013, 128(1):88–91.
21. Dowrick C. *Beyond depression: a new approach to understanding and management.* Oxford: Oxford University Press, 2009.
22. Magpie Research Group. The nature and prevalence of psychological problems in New Zealand primary healthcare: a report on mental health and general practice investigation (MAGPIE). *NZ Med J* 2003, 116:1171–1185.
23. Goldberg D, Klinkman M. Primary health care and the ICD-11. *Die Psychiatrie* 2013, 10 (1):33–37.
24. Lieberman JA, 3rd, Stuart MR. The BATHE method: incorporating counseling and psychotherapy into the everyday management of patients. *Prim Care Companion J Clin Psychiatry* 1999, 1(2):35–38.
25. Robertson K. Active listening: more than just paying attention. *Aust Fam Physician* 2005, 34(12):1053–1055.
26. Freeman TR. *McWhinney's textbook of family medicine.* 4th edition. Oxford: Oxford University Press, 2016.

27. Strosahl K, Robinson P, Gustavsson T. *Brief interventions for radical change: principles and practice of focussed acceptance and commitment therapy*. Oakland, CA: New Harbinger Publications, 2012.

28. Kroenke K, Spitzer RL, Williams JB, et al. Physical symptoms in primary care: predictors of psychiatric disorders and functional impairment. *Arch Fam Med* 1994, 3(9):774–779.

29. Arroll B, Goodyear-Smith F, Kerse N, et al. Effect of the addition of a "help" question to two screening questions on specificity for diagnosis of depression in general practice: diagnostic validity study. *BMJ* 2005, 331(7521):884. doi: 10.1136/bmj.38607.464537.7C.

30. Kroenke K, Spitzer RL. The PHQ-9: a new depression diagnostic and severity measure. *Psychiatr Ann* 2002, 32:509–521.

31. Pirkis J, Burgess P. Suicide and recency of health care contacts: a systematic review. *Br J Psychiatry* 1998, 173:462–474.

32. The National Institute for Health and Care Excellence. Depression in adults: recognition and management. nice.org.uk/guidance/cg90 updated 2016.

33. Hughes T, Cardno A, West R, et al. Unrecognised bipolar disorder among UK primary care patients prescribed antidepressants: an observational study. *Br J Gen Pract* 2016, 66(643):e71-717. doi: 10.3399/bjgp16X683437.

34. Arroll B, Moir F, Kendrick T. Effective management of depression in primary care: a review of the literature. *BJGP Open* 2017, 1(2): pii: BJGP-2016-0125.

35. Gilbody S, Richards D, Barkham M. Diagnosing depression in primary care using self-completed instruments: UK validation of PHQ-9 and CORE-OM. *Br J Gen Pract* 2007, 57(541):650–652.

36. Chin WY, Chan KT, Lam CL, et al. 12-Month naturalistic outcomes of depressive disorders in Hong Kong's primary care. *Fam Pract* 2015, 32(3):288–296. doi: 10.1093/fampra/cmv009.

37. Balint M. *The doctor, his patient and the illness*. London: Churchill Livingstone, 1957.

38. National Institute for Health and Care Excellence (NICE). *Depression in adults: recognition and management (CG90)*. London, 2009.

39. Donker T, Griffiths KM, Cuijpers P, et al. Psychoeducation for depression, anxiety and psychological distress: a meta-analysis. *BMC Med* 2009, 7:79. doi: 10.1186/1741-7015-7-79.

40. Bass J, Neugebauer R, Clougherty KF, et al. Group interpersonal psychotherapy for depression in rural Uganda: 6-month outcomes: randomised controlled trial. *Br J Psychiatry* 2006, 188:567–573. doi: 10.1192/bjp.188.6.567.

41. Cooney G, Dwan K, Mead G. Exercise for depression. *JAMA* 2014, 311(23):2432–2433.

42. Hallgren M, Vancampfort D, Stubbs B. Exercise is medicine for depression: even when the "pill" is small (letter). *Neuropsychiatr Dis Treat* 2016, 12:2715–2721.

43. Harris R. *ACT made simple. An easy-to-read primer on acceptance and commitment therapy*. Oakland, CA: New Harbinger Publications, 2009.

44. Fournier JC, DeRubeis RJ, Hollon SD, et al. Antidepressant drug effects and depression severity: a patient-level meta-analysis. *JAMA* 2010, 303(1):47–53.

45. Stone M, Kalaria S, Richardville K, et al. Components and trends in treatment effects in randomized placebo-controlled trials in major depressive disorder from 1979–2016. American Society of Clinical Psychopharmacology. Miami 2018.

46. Warner CH, Bobo W, Warner C, et al. Antidepressant discontinuation syndrome. *Am Fam Physician* 2006, 74(3):449–456.

47. Lewis G, Duffy L, Ades A, et al. The clinical effectiveness of sertraline in primary care and the role of depression severity and duration (PANDA): a pragmatic, double-blind,

placebo-controlled randomised trial. *Lancet Psychiatry* 2019, doi: 10.1016/S2215-0366(19)30366-9 [published Online First: 2019/09/24].

48. Dowrick C, Frances A. Medicalising unhappiness: new classification of depression risks more patients being put on drug treatment from which they will not benefit. *BMJ* 2013, 347(7):f7140.

49. Hunkeler E, Merseman JF, Hargreaves WA, et al. Efficacy of nurse telehealth care and peer support in augmenting treatment of depression in primary care. *Arch Fam Med* 2000, 9:700–708.

50. Gensichen J, Guethlin C, Sarmand N, et al. Patients' perspectives on depression case management in general practice: a qualitative study. *Patient Educ Couns* 2012, 86(1):114–119. doi: 10.1016/j.pec.2011.02.020.

51. McKall K. An insider's guide to depression. *BMJ* 2001, 323:1011.

Chapter 3

# NON-DRUG INTERVENTIONS FOR COMMON MENTAL HEALTH PROBLEMS

Weng Yee Chin

# Key points

1. Demonstrate active listening and clinical interpersonal skills to show warmth, interest, respect, empathy and support.
2. Effectively assess a patient's psychosocial status, e.g. using the BATHE technique.
3. Provide psychoeducation.
4. Teach relaxation and stress management techniques.
5. Incorporate principles of behavioural activation into the management plan.
6. Support patients in using internet-based psychological treatments.
7. Empower patients to become better problem solvers.

# Introduction

Common mental health disorders, such as depression and anxiety, affect up to 15% of the population at any one time.[1] The 2010 Global Burden of Disease study found that major depressive disorders accounted for 8.2% of global years lived with disability (YLD) making it the second leading cause of YLDs after cardiovascular disease.[2] To date, the most common method used to manage common mental health disorders in primary care has been with psychotropic medications[3] despite the fact that non-pharmacological treatments are often preferred by patients[1] and have been shown to be effective.[4] Referral of patients for psychological services can be difficult because of limited access to qualified therapists and patient barriers such as time and stigma.[5] Methods of providing psychological treatments that are less resource intensive, accessible, affordable and non-stigmatising to patients are of great importance to primary care.[6]

The primary care setting is the point of entry for most people into the health system. Family doctors are well placed to deliver mental health interventions due to the longitudinal relationship and trust they have with patients and families, their ability to respond to undifferentiated problems, the use of a bio-psychosocial model and their ability to integrate care of mental conditions with physical conditions.[7]

Mental health presentations most frequently encountered by family doctors include generic psychosocial distress, grief, bereavement, sub-threshold mood symptoms, reactive disorders, mild to moderate unipolar depressive disorders and anxiety disorders, which can be of sufficient severity to impair daily functioning or health-related quality of life. Such presentations may account for as much as 30% of consultations in primary care.[8] In many primary care settings, usual care for depression and anxiety typically involves empathic listening, provision of some informal supportive counselling, prescription of psychotropic medications (usually antidepressants), a medical certificate and/or a referral to a mental health service.[9] Evidence from several meta-analyses have found that the effectiveness of antidepressants over placebo appears to be minimal or non-existent in mild or moderate depression, but may be more substantial in patients with very severe depression.[10] The risk-benefit ratio for antidepressants is therefore reasonably poor for most primary care patients who tend to have mild to moderate symptoms when weighed against the adverse drug effects associated with tolerability and withdrawal.[10] NICE guidelines currently advise avoiding drug treatment unless there is a past history of moderate or severe depression that persists after other interventions have been trialled, or subthreshold symptoms that have been present for a long period typically at least two years.[11]

Non-drug interventions for common mental health problems can take a variety of forms ranging from supportive and empathic clinical interpersonal communication techniques and low intensity psychosocial interventions that can be delivered by any family doctor, to more intensive psychological therapies provided by trained therapists. The aim of this chapter is to help raise awareness of the role of non-drug interventions (NDIs) in managing common mental health disorders, and to encourage family doctors to incorporate these evidence-based treatments into their routine practice.

# Recommendations on the types of skills that family doctors need

### 1. Clinical interpersonal skills

Interpersonal skills are an important and integral part of the practice of good medicine. There is a large body of evidence supporting the value of core attributes and skills such as showing empathy,[12-14] compassion,[15] and being able to provide patient support. These competencies are relevant not only for reducing patient distress, but studies have also found that doctors who possess and demonstrate such skills are more effective. Patients have better faith in their doctors and are more willing to adhere to their treatments ultimately resulting in better mental and physical wellbeing.[16,17] Techniques such as the Cambridge–Calgary method[18] which emphasises active listening skills and the BATHE technique[19,20] as a method for assessing a patient's psychosocial status have been shown to result in more effective GP consultations and increased patient satisfaction.[18,21]

Studies have found that formal training of doctors and medical students is effective.[18] An educational programme in mindful communication was found to enhance empathy and patient-centred care, and reduce burnout;[22] family physicians taking part reported enhanced ability to listen deeply to patients' concerns and develop their own adaptive reserves.[23] Empathy training modules in postgraduate medical education have been shown to significantly impact empathy scores as rated by patients.[24]

## Recommended competencies

Be able to demonstrate active listening and clinical interpersonal skills to show warmth, interest, respect, empathy and non-judgmental support.[21]

- Attentive body language: facial expressions, eye contact, gestures to show engagement and interest;
- Following skills: open-ended questions to facilitate the patient to tell their story, attentive silences, facilitative responses, picking up on cues;
- Reflecting skills: paraphrasing, summarising or repeating back what has been said to clarify and show understanding, reflect back feelings.

Be able to effectively assess a patient's psychosocial status, e.g. using the BATHE technique.[19]

- Background: e.g. "What's going on in your life?"; "Tell me what has been happening?"
- Affect: e.g. "How does that make you feel?"; "How has that affected you?"
- Trouble: e.g. "What troubles you about this?"; "What bothers you the most about the situation?"
- Handling: e.g. "How are you handling that?"; "How have you been managing this problem?"
- Empathy: Instil hope by expressing your understanding of what the patient is going through e.g. "I imagine that could be/may be difficult"; "You seem to be going through a lot."

## 2. Skills in delivering low intensity psychosocial interventions

Low intensity psychological interventions refer to interventions that do not rely on mental health specialists and may consist of modified, brief evidence-based therapies including guided self-help or e-mental health.[25] They tend to be trans-diagnostic (can be used for any type of common mental health disorder) with a primary focus on enhancing patients' self-efficacy.[26] Evidence-based interventions include psychoeducation, stress management and relaxation techniques, behavioural activation, cognitive behavioural therapy (either in individual or group format) and problem-solving therapy. Low intensity psychosocial skills training can feasibly be incorporated into medical school curricula even when curriculum time is limited.[27]

### 2.1. Psychoeducation

**Description**

Psychoeducation refers to any educational intervention offered to individuals (and their families) to help empower them to improve their health. Psycho-education can help to reduce stigma, self-blame and barriers to treatment. The key goals of psychoeducation are:

- Knowledge transfer (e.g. pathophysiology or the cause of the illness, education about treatments);
- Promote understanding (e.g. to understand what can make things worse or better);
- Support treatment (e.g. to enhance compliance);
- Promote self-help (e.g. what to do if a crisis occurs).

**Evidence**

A meta-analysis found that brief psychoeducational interventions for depression and psychological distress can reduce symptoms and are easy to implement as an initial intervention for psychological distress or depression in primary care.[28] Studies have found that psychoeducation can help to prevent and reduce the risk of relapse of depression.[28,29]

Current evidence suggests that whilst the quality of psychoeducation provided is important, the method of delivery appears to be less important (e.g. patient information leaflets, face-to-face discussion, group-based classes).[28] This means that even in a busy GP setting, doctors can provide psychoeducation by promoting individualised self-help (e.g. by referring patients to books or websites or providing patient education leaflets) or refer patients to group psychoeducation classes.

**Recommended skills**

- Be able to provide psychoeducation for depression, anxiety and panic attacks – pathophysiology, effect on health and treatments;
- Be able to explain the sleep cycle and its effect on mental health;
- Be able to provide instructions on sleep hygiene.

### 2.2. Stress management and relaxation techniques

**Description**

Stress, especially that relating to work, is a common trigger for health problems presenting to primary care.[30] There is a body of research connecting stress to physical health problems such as cardiovascular disease, metabolic syndrome, obesity, weakened immunity and infertility through disturbances of the hypothalamic-pituitary axis and increased cortisol levels, as well as to mental illnesses such as depression.[31,32] Given the negative impact of stress, it is important for family doctors to be familiar with commonly used stress management and relaxation techniques and to be able to teach them to their patients.

**Evidence**

Stress management techniques can reduce psychological distress. Examples include slow breathing or diaphragmatic breathing exercises, progressive muscle relaxation, guided imagery or guided meditation and mindfulness-based stress reduction (MBSR).[33] A review paper on stress reduction techniques found that they can improve the quality of life of patients and contribute to the reduction of physical and psychological symptoms, and that the same techniques can be therapeutic for health care providers and help to enhance their interactions with patients.[33] A recent Dutch pilot study of mindfulness-based stress reduction for GPs has found positive effects on dedication, mindfulness and compassion.[34] Training intensity for these techniques can range from a half-day session to 8–12 week courses.

**Recommended skills**

- Be able to teach slow breathing exercises;
- Be able to teach progressive muscle relaxation;
- Be able to promote and support patients to practice guided relaxation, meditation and/or mindfulness-based interventions.

## 2.3. Behavioural activation

**Description**

Behavioural activation is a therapeutic process that emphasises planned activities which help to increase behaviours that are likely to produce improvements in thoughts, mood, and overall quality of life.[35] The aim of behavioural activation is to structure in positive distractions and mood improving activities. These activities aim to increase pleasurable activities, enhance social interactions, promote better sleep and improve self-esteem. It helps to enhance mood by reducing mood-worsening rumination whilst promoting positive reinforcing thoughts and feelings.[35]

**Evidence**

Behavioural activation is targeted predominantly at patients who may be depressed, socially withdrawn or have poor self-esteem.[36,37] This may be particularly important in the elderly who are prone to social isolation due to physical illness.[38] There is some evidence that it may also be effective for anxiety.[39] Exercise (on its own or incorporated into an activity plan) should also be promoted routinely by GPs. A Cochrane review found that exercise is moderately more effective than a control intervention for reducing symptoms of depression, and as effective as psychological or pharmacological treatments.[40] A 2016 trial found that exercise is beneficial for depression even when it is light (yoga and stretching) as opposed to moderate and vigorous and when conducted once per week.[41] Furthermore, there can be cardiovascular and metabolic benefits for patients with depression.

Incorporating an activity plan is feasible in a routine GP consultation.[42] A doctor can help guide their patient to draw up a schedule of planned activities. These activities should be negotiated using a patient-centred approach, to enhance compliance and effectiveness in alleviating mood symptoms. Activities could include day-to-day essentials (bathing, shopping, eating and sleeping) with the incorporation of social activities (e.g. lunch with a friend), pleasurable activities (e.g. hiking, watching a movie) and activities that can promote self-esteem (e.g. gardening, volunteer work). Patients need to be encouraged to remain engaged and active even if they do not feel like doing it.

**Recommended skills**

- Be able to negotiate with the patient to construct a patient-centred activity plan;
- Be able to encourage and motivate a patient to keep engaged in pleasurable activities and activities that can improve self-esteem and self-efficacy;
- Be able to motivate patients to keep physically active;
- Be able to facilitate patients to strengthen their social supports.

### 2.4. Internet-based psychological treatments, e.g. iCBT

In many countries, computer-based therapies such as internet-delivered cognitive behavioural therapy (iCBT) is gaining significant attention as a way to scale up the delivery of psychological services and has been found to be as effective as traditional CBT. A 2012 review on internet-based psychological treatments found that iCBT interventions are effective and provide an important alternative to face-to-face psychological treatments, but that guided iCBT treatments (either with the GP or an allied health staff) are more effective than unguided treatments. Contact before and/or after the treatment can enhance both guided and unguided iCBT.[43]

**Recommended skills**

- Be able to facilitate and support patients using guided internet-based psychological therapies such as iCBT.

Free examples of iCBT:

- Mood gym: https://moodgym.anu.edu.au/welcome

### 2.5. Problem-solving therapy (PST)

**Description**

Problem-solving therapy (PST) is a focused psychological intervention that helps patients to develop problem-solving skills to address life problems associated with psychological and somatic symptoms. It can help various psychological problems including depression, anxiety and sleep disturbance. The aim is to empower the patient to identify and solve their own problems by guiding them through the problem-solving process in a structured, sequential way. An abbreviated version has been developed for use in primary care that can be delivered over a series of four to six 15–30 minute consultations.[44]

### Evidence

PST has been shown to be as effective as antidepressant medication for major depression in improving symptoms and social functioning when provided by appropriately skilled GPs.[45] Primary care doctors and nurses can learn to deliver PST by doing a short training programme.[46]

### Recommended skills

- Be able to facilitate patients to identify specific life problems associated with psychological and/or somatic symptoms;
- Be able to guide patients to set specific, achievable goal/s;
- Be able to assist patients to brainstorm possible solutions and weigh up their pros and cons;
- Be able to empower patients to decide on and implement a plan of action, and to review the outcomes.

## Implications for service delivery

The WHO Mental Health Gap Action Programme (mhGAP) have developed and evaluated a set of training manuals for scalable psychological interventions to help build mental health capacity. These manuals are intended for training non-specialised health workers with no prior mental health qualifications. These interventions are particularly relevant for settings where access to psychological services is limited and in great need such as in communities affected by adversity.[47] They currently include:

- **mhGAP Intervention Guide – Version 2.0**: for mental, neurological and substance use disorders in non-specialised health settings. www.who.int/mental_health/mhgap/mhGAP_intervention_guide_02/en/

- **Thinking healthy**: a manual for psychosocial management of perinatal depression.[48] www.who.int/mental_health/maternal-child/thinking_healthy/en/
- **Problem Management Plus (PM+)**: PM+ is for adults suffering from symptoms of common mental health problems (e.g. depression, anxiety, stress or grief), as well as self-identified practical problems (e.g. unemployment, interpersonal conflict). It uses a trans-diagnostic approach that can be very useful in primary care where many patients present with comorbidity or no specified diagnosis. PM+ integrates problem-solving and behavioural treatment techniques with a strong emphasis on behavioural (as opposed to cognitive) techniques, as these are easier to teach and learn.[49] www.who.int/mental_health/emergencies/problem_management_plus/en/
- **Guidance on group interpersonal therapy (IPT)**: WHO recommends interpersonal therapy (IPT) as a first line treatment for depression. WHO guidance on use of IPT uses an eight session group protocol for use by supervised facilitators who may not have received previous training in mental health.[50] www.who.int/mental_health/mhgap/interpersonal_therapy/en/

## The Collaborative Care Model for delivery of mental health services in primary care

Over the past decade, the Collaborative Care Model as originally described by Katon and colleagues[51] has been shown to improve patient outcomes, save money, and reduce stigma related to mental health. Collaborative Care operationalises the principles of Wagner's Chronic Care Model[52] to improve access to evidence-based mental health treatments for primary care patients. It helps to normalise and de-stigmatise treatments for behavioural health disorders and enhances service access for patients. In this integrated team-based, stepped care approach, patients are managed by a primary care clinician and a case manager. A specialist psychiatrist liaises usually via the case manager to provide advice on diagnosis and treatment when first line treatments are not effective. Training in collaborative/integrated care can help optimise the skill mix to enhance the outcomes for mental health problems in primary care.[53] The American Psychiatric Association/Academy of Psychosomatic Medicine has produced a report summarising the evidence on how to implement Collaborative Care Model for mental health into primary care.[54]

# Educational material

### Case study

Mr. P, aged 49 years, presents with two months of fatigue and tiredness. He claims that this is unlike him as he is usually very energetic and motivated. He tells you that he thinks his is "just fatigued from working long hours lately". You do not know him well as it has been a few years since you last saw him.

*What should you do next?*

- Ask him why he has waited so long to see a doctor about this problem OR
- Praise him for taking time out of his busy schedule to talk about his health.

Studies have shown that men have much lower rates of seeking medical attention than women. This lower help-seeking pattern has been observed across a range of problems including general physical health, psychosocial health and substance use. Failing to seek help can lead to delayed treatment and contribute to poorer health outcomes, and greater personal and health system burdens.

However, it is not helpful to criticise a patient for seeking help in this way. Providing affirmation and positive reinforcement for positive help-seeking behaviours can help normalise medical consultations for men allowing them to build trust with medical professionals and be more inclined to be proactive to seek help when issues arise. Engaging the patient by showing that you are listening empathically helps to build the doctor–patient therapeutic alliance. You can use the BATHE technique to further explore the patient's psychosocial situation and their coping skills.

His wife is your patient, and you know from her that they have three teenage sons and that he has recently left his work in an insurance company to work for an NGO.

He is a non-smoker but drinks 3–4 glasses of wine/beer per day. He takes no regular medications but has been taking the occasional paracetamol for headaches. He has no significant past medical or family history.

Work has been stressful lately due to a series of deadlines, but he still finds his work meaningful.

His marital relationship is good except however he admits he has had very little interest in sex. His sons have been rebellious, and he is finding fathering teenagers rather challenging. He is worried about money as he is earning less than before.

*What is his main problem?*
- Physiological fatigue and undifferentiated psychological distress OR
- Mixed anxiety and depression disorder.

Mr. P is undergoing several life adjustments including a new career and work environment, a new stage in his family's life cycle, and a lower household income. With adjustment comes stress as the individual learns to adapt to their changed circumstances. The impact of these changes will depend in part on the amount of burden imposed and in part on their ability to cope. Stress and fatigue will occur when the burden outweighs their ability to cope.

According to ICD-10, mixed anxiety and depressive disorder (MADD) is characterised by co-existing, sub-syndromic symptoms of anxiety and depression where neither dominate, but severe enough to justify a psychiatric diagnosis. It is associated with a similar degree of distress, impairment to daily functioning, and reduction in health-related quality of life as major depressive or anxiety disorders. Mr P does not fulfil the criteria for this diagnosis.

On further questioning, he reports that his appetite is good, but he "stress eats" and has gained weight recently. Sleep has been a problem as he goes to bed late and it takes him a while to wind down. He denies feeling depressed but knows he tends to be a bit of a "worrier".

His BP is 140/90 and BMI is 29; all other physical examinations are normal.

*How should his problems be managed?*
- Arrange investigations to rule out cancer or anaemia and a follow-up after the results are available to discuss them OR
- Explain the reason for his fatigue and discuss the patient's preferred treatment options with a follow-up to assess his response to treatment.

Fatigue is a commonly encountered presenting symptom in primary care. Investigations can be useful to exclude disease and may help to reassure patients who are concerned about specific diagnoses, but typically, there is a low rate for identifying underlying disease. Investigations are warranted in those who have not recovered after one month, whose initial presentation is atypical, or where "red flag" symptoms or signs are present.

Explain to the patient that that he has the common problem of undifferentiated fatigue. Contributing factors include lifestyle stress and anxiety resulting from his heavy workload, financial pressures, home pressures, and insufficient rest and exercise. This has all contributed to his lack of energy, increase in weight, reduced libido and mild hypertension.

Praise his strong work ethic and reassure him that his outlook is good if he follows sensible lifestyle advice such as a regular sleep routine (sleep hygiene), the introduction of some physical activity which he enjoys (exercise prescription), and scheduling some time to do things that he enjoys (behavioural activation).

He shows some indicators that place him at risk of depression, so it is important to monitor this. Schedule the patient to return for a follow-up to monitor BP, weight and mood.

# Multiple choice questions

1. Your patient is a 49-year-old male who presents with a two-month history of fatigue and difficulty concentrating at work. Which of the following describes a core symptom of depression?

   a. Falls asleep during meetings at work.
   b. Has difficulty waking up in time for work.
   c. Regularly works until late at night.
   d. Has lost interest in his work.

2. Your patient is a 49-year-old male who presents complaining of fatigue and poor sleep. When would sleep hygiene education be the most appropriate sleep intervention?

   a. Frequent night-time waking associated with snoring and apnoeic episodes.
   b. Low mood, loss of interest and early morning wakening.
   c. Irregular sleep patterns due to daytime napping and staying up late watching TV.
   d. Ruminating thoughts keeping him awake at night.

3. Your patient is a 49-year-old male who presents with mild depressive symptoms including low mood, poor self-esteem

and social withdrawal. How should you introduce behavioural activation?

a. Tell him that he needs to get out more to socialise.

b. Recommend that he signs up to a six month membership at a nearby gym.

c. Provide him with some pamphlets of local NGOs where he can do some volunteer work.

d. Ask him to identify activities that he enjoys and encourage him to do it even if he doesn't feel like doing it.

4. Your patient is a 49-year-old male who presents with episodes of breathlessness and palpitations that you diagnose as panic attacks. What is the most appropriate first line non-drug intervention for patients presenting with panic attacks?

a. Psychoeducation.

b. Relaxation techniques.

c. Behavioural activation.

d. iCBT.

You will find the answers to these MCQs on page 171.

# Further reading and e-resources

**Clinical interpersonal skills**

| | |
|---|---|
| Active listening | www.racgp.org.au/afpbackissues/2005/200512/200512robinson.pdf |
| BATHE technique | http://primhe.org.uk/documents/relavent_docs/BATHE_technique.pdf |
| Communication skills | https://www.each.eu/teaching/resources/ |

**Psychoeducation**

| | |
|---|---|
| Depression | www.cci.health.wa.gov.au/Resources/For-Clinicians/Depression |
| | www.racgp.org.au/afp/2013/april/bibliotherapy-for-depression/ |
| Panic attacks | www.cci.health.wa.gov.au/Resources/For-Clinicians/Anxiety |
| Sleep | https://sleep.org/ |
| | https://sleepfoundation.org/sleep-topics/sleep-hygiene |
| iCBT | www.racgp.org.au/afp/2013/november/cbt/ |

| | MoodGYM (https://moodgym.anu.edu.au/welcome) is a free online training programme developed by the Centre for Mental Health Research, Australian National University. It uses CBT and interpersonal therapy. MoodGYM is available in several languages. |
|---|---|
| **Relaxation exercises** | |
| Slow breathing | www.cci.health.wa.gov.au/Resources/Looking-After-Yourself/Other-Resources<br>www.youtube.com/watch?v=aN05yXFbwI0 (YouTube video) |
| Progressive muscle relaxation | www.cci.health.wa.gov.au/docs/ACF3C8D.pdf |
| **Behavioural activation** | |
| Activity scheduling | www.cci.health.wa.gov.au/Resources/For-Clinicians/Depression<br>http://psychologytools.com/task-planning-and-achievement-record.html |
| Exercise prescription | www.move.va.gov/docs/Resources/CHPPM_How_To_Write_And_Exercise_Prescription.pdf |
| **Problem solving therapy** | www.racgp.org.au/afp/2012/september/problem-solving-therapy/#16 |
| **Training manuals and guidelines** | |
| mhGAP Intervention Guide – Version 2.0 | www.who.int/mental_health/mhgap/mhGAP_intervention_guide_02/en/ |
| Thinking healthy | www.who.int/mental_health/maternal-child/thinking_healthy/en/ |
| Problem Management Plus (PM+) | www.who.int/mental_health/emergencies/problem_management_plus/en/ |
| Interpersonal therapy | www.who.int/mental_health/mhgap/interpersonal_therapy/en/ |
| Problem-solving therapy | Weel-Baumgarten, E. van, Mynors-Wallis, L., Jané-Llopis, E., & Anderson, P. (2005). A training manual for prevention of mental illness: managing emotional symptoms and problems in primary care. Nijmegen: Radboud University of Nijmegen. http://uwaims.org/files/pst/PST-PC_Manual.pdf |
| Collaborative Care Model | American Psychiatric Association/Academy of Psychosomatic Medicine. Dissemination of integrated care within adult primary care settings: the collaborative care model 2016. www.psychiatry.org/File%20Library/Psychiatrists/Practice/Professional-Topics/Integrated-Care/APA-APM-Dissemination-Integrated-Care-Report.pdf |

Atención a Las Personas con Malestar Emocional: Relacionado con Condicionantes Sociales en Atención Primaria de Salud (in Spanish)
https://consaludmental.org/publicaciones/Atencion-personas-malestar-emocional.pdf

# References

1. National Collaborating Centre for Mental Health (Great Britain), National Institute for Health, Clinical Excellence (Great Britain), British Psychological Society and Royal College of Psychiatrists, 2011. *Common mental health disorders: identification and pathways to care* (Vol. 123). RCPsych Publications.
2. Ferrari AJ, Charlson FJ, Norman RE, et al. Burden of depressive disorders by country, sex, age, and year: findings from the global burden of disease study 2010. *PLoS Med* 2013, 10(11):e1001547.
3. Young AS, Klap R, Sherbourne CD, et al. The quality of care for depressive and anxiety disorders in the United States. *Arch Gen Psychiatr* 2001, 58(1):55–61.
4. Farah WH, Alsawas M, Mainou M, et al. Non-pharmacological treatment of depression: a systematic review and evidence map. *BMJ Evidence Based Medicine* 2016, 21(6):214–21. ebmed-2016-110522.
5. Swift JK, Greenberg RP. Premature discontinuation in adult psychotherapy: a meta-analysis. *J Consult Clin Psychol* 2012, Aug 80(4):547.
6. Mohr DC, Ho J, Duffecy J, et al. Perceived barriers to psychological treatments and their relationship to depression. *J Clinical Psychol* 2010, 66(4):394–409.
7. Culpepper L. The active management of depression. *J Fam Practice* 2002, Sep 51(9):769–77.
8. Wittchen H-U, Jacobi F. Size and burden of mental disorders in Europe: a critical review and appraisal of 27 studies. *Eur Neuropsychopharm* 2005, 15(4):357–76.
9. Chin WY, Chan KT, Lam CL, et al. Detection and management of depression in adult primary care patients in Hong Kong: a cross-sectional survey conducted by a primary care practice-based research network. *BMC Fam Pract* 2014, 15(1):30.
10. Arroll B, Chin W, Matris W, et al. Antidepressants for treatment of depression in primary care: a systematic review and meta-analysis. *J Prim Health Care* 2016, 8(4):325–34.
11. National Collaborating Centre for Mental Health (UK). *Depression: the treatment and management of depression in adults* (updated edition). Leicester (UK), British Psychological Society 2010. (NICE Clinical Guidelines, No. 90).
12. van Osch M, Sep M, van Vliet LM, et al. Reducing patients' anxiety and uncertainty, and improving recall in bad news consultations. *Health Psychol* 2014, 33(11):1382–90.
13. Mercer SW, Higgins M, Bikker AM, et al. General practitioners' empathy and health outcomes: a prospective observational study of consultations in areas of high and low deprivation. *Ann Fam Med* 2016, 14(2):117–24.
14. Bensing JM, Verheul W. The silent healer: the role of communication in placebo effects. *Pat Educ Counsel* 2010, 80(3):293–99.
15. Jani BD, Blane DN, Mercer SW. The role of empathy in therapy and the physician-patient relationship. *Res Complemen Med* 2012, 19(5):252–57.
16. van Os TW, van Den Brink RH, Tiemens BG, et al. Communicative skills of general practitioners augment the effectiveness of guideline-based depression treatment. *J Aff Disord* 2005, 84(1):43–51.
17. Del Canale S, Louis DZ, Maio V, et al. The relationship between physician empathy and disease complications: an empirical study of primary care physicians and their diabetic patients in Parma, Italy. *Acad Med* 2012, 87(9):1243–49.
18. Silverman J, Kurtz S, Draper J. *Skills for communicating with patients*. 3rd edn. Boca Raton, CRC Press 2013.

19. Leiblum SR, Schnall E, Seehuus M, et al. To BATHE or not to BATHE: patient satisfaction with visits to their family physician. Fam Med 2008, 40(6):407.

20. Searight HR. Efficient counseling techniques for the primary care physician. *Prim Care; Clinics in Office Practice* 2007, Sep 34(3):551–70.

21. Robertson K. Active listening: more than just paying attention. *Aus Fam Physician* 2005, 34(12):1053.

22. Krasner MS, Epstein RM, Beckman H, et al. Association of an educational program in mindful communication with burnout, empathy, and attitudes among primary care physicians. *JAMA* 2009, 302(12):1284–93.

23. Beckman HB, Wendland M, Mooney C, et al. The impact of a program in mindful communication on primary care physicians. *Acad Med* 2012, 87(6):815–19.

24. Riess H, Kelley JM, Bailey RW, et al. Empathy training for resident physicians: a randomized controlled trial of a neuroscience-informed curriculum. *J Gen Int Med* 2012, 27(10):1280–86.

25. Rodgers M, Asaria M, Walker S, et al. The clinical effectiveness and cost-effectiveness of low-intensity psychological interventions for the secondary prevention of relapse after depression: a systematic review. *Health Technol Assess* 2012, May 16(28):1–130.

26. Cape J, Whittington C, Buszewicz M, et al. Brief psychological therapies for anxiety and depression in primary care: meta-analysis and meta-regression. *BMC Medicine* 2010, 8(1):38.

27. Chin W-Y, Lam C, Wong C. Development of a tool to assess the impact of a brief counseling curriculum: validation of the Attitudes To Psychological Interventions and Counseling in Primary Care (APIC-PC) survey. *Pat Educ Counsel* 2011, 85(3):481–86.

28. Donker T, Griffiths KM, Cuijpers P, et al. Psychoeducation for depression, anxiety and psychological distress: a meta-analysis. *BMC Medicine* 2009, 7(1):79.

29. Cuijpers P, Andersson G, Donker T, et al. Psychological treatment of depression: results of a series of meta-analyses. *Nordic J Psychiatr* 2011, 65(6):354–64.

30. Mental health: facing the challenges, building solutions. Report from the WHO European Ministerial Conference on Mental Health, Helsinki, Finland, January 2005. World Health Organization.

31. McEwen BS. Central effects of stress hormones in health and disease: understanding the protective and damaging effects of stress and stress mediators. *Eur J Pharmacol* 2008, 583(2):174–85.

32. Pedersen A, Zachariae R, Bovbjerg DH. Influence of psychological stress on upper respiratory infection: a meta-analysis of prospective studies. *Psychosom Med* 2010, 72(8):823–32.

33. Varvogli L, Darviri C. Stress management techniques: evidence-based procedures that reduce stress and promote health. *Health Sci J* 2011, Apr 5(2):74.

34. Verweij H, Waumans RC, Smeijers D, et al. Mindfulness-based stress reduction for GPs: results of a controlled mixed methods pilot study in Dutch primary care. *Br J Gen Pract* 2016, 66(643):e99-e105.

35. Hopko DR, Lejuez C, Ruggiero KJ, et al. Contemporary behavioral activation treatments for depression: procedures, principles, and progress. *Clin Pychol Rev* 2003, 23 (5):699–717.

36. Mazzucchelli T, Kane R, Rees C. Behavioral activation treatments for depression in adults: a meta-analysis and review. *Clin Psychol Sci Practice* 2009, 16(4):383–411.

37. Ekers D, Webster L, Van Straten A, et al. Behavioural activation for depression: an update of meta-analysis of effectiveness and sub group analysis. *PLOS One* 2014, 9(6): e100100.

38. Hunkeler EM, Katon W, Tang L, et al. Long term outcomes from the IMPACT randomised trial for depressed elderly patients in primary care. *BMJ* 2006, 332:259–63.

39. Hopko DR, Robertson S, Lejuez C. Behavioral activation for anxiety disorders. *Behavior Analyst Today* 2006, 7(2):212.

40. Cooney G, Dwan K, Mead G. Exercise for depression. *JAMA* 2014, 311(23):2432–33.

41. Hallgren M, Vancampfort D, Stubbs B. Exercise is medicine for depression: even when the "pill" is small (letter). *Neuropsychiatr Dis Treat* 2016, 12:2715–21.

42. Cuijpers P, Van Straten A, Warmerdam L. Behavioral activation treatments of depression: a meta-analysis. *Clin Psychol Rev* 2007, 27(3):318–26.

43. Johansson R, Andersson G. Internet-based psychological treatments for depression. *Expert Rev Neurother* 2012, 12(7):861–70.

44. Mynors-Wallis L. *Problem-solving treatment for anxiety and depression: a practical guide*. Oxford, Oxford University Press 2005.

45. Mynors-Wallis LM, Gath DH, Day A, et al. Randomised controlled trial of problem solving treatment, antidepressant medication, and combined treatment for major depression in primary care. *Br Med J* 2000, 320:26–30.

46. van Weel-Baumgarten E, Jane-Liopis E, Mynors-Wallis L, et al. Prevention of mental illness in primary care. *Eur J Gen Practice* 2005, 11(3–4):92–93.

47. World Health Organization. Scalable psychological interventions for people in communities affected by adversity: a new area of mental health and psychosocial work at WHO. 2017.

48. World Health Organization. Thinking healthy: a manual for psychosocial management of perinatal depression, WHO generic field-trial version 1.0, 2015.

49. Dawson KS, Bryant RA, Harper M, et al. Problem Management Plus (PM+): a WHO transdiagnostic psychological intervention for common mental health problems. *World Psychiatry* 2015, 14(3):354–57.

50. Bass J, Neugebauer R, Clougherty KF, et al. Group interpersonal psychotherapy for depression in rural Uganda: 6-month outcomes: randomised controlled trial. *Br J Psychiatry* 2006, 188:567–73.

51. Katon WJ, Seelig M, Katon WJ, et al. Population-based care of depression: team care approaches to improving outcomes. *J Occup Environ Med* 2008, 50(4):459–67.

52. Wagner E, Austin B, Von Korff M. Improving outcomes in chronic illness. *Manag Care Q* 1996, 4(2):12–25.

53. Funk M, Ivbijaro G. *Integrating mental health into primary care: a global perspective*. Geneva, WONCA-WHO 2008.

54. Vanderlip ER, Rundell J, Avery M, Alter C, Engel C, Fortney J, Williams M. *Dissemination of integrated care within adult primary care settings: the collaborative care model*. Washington DC, American Psychiatric Association and Academy of Psychosomatic Medicine 2016.

Chapter 4

# MEDICALLY UNEXPLAINED SYMPTOMS

Tim olde Hartman, Christopher Dowrick, Cindy L K Lam, Sandra Fortes, David Clarke and Jinan Usta

# Key points

1. Medically unexplained symptoms (MUS) are physical symptoms that have existed for several weeks, for which adequate medical examination or investigation have not revealed any medical condition that sufficiently explains the symptoms.
2. MUS is not a diagnosis, but an ongoing working hypothesis.
3. MUS can be seen as a continuum from mild to severe.
4. The causes of MUS can be categorized into predisposing, precipitating and perpetuating factors and can be linked to the biopsychosocial model.
5. Family doctors can set a working hypothesis of MUS after a broad biopsychosocial exploration.
6. Family doctors should focus on the doctor–patient relationship and doctor–patient communication.
7. Family doctors should provide a targeted and tangible explanation.
8. Family doctors should focus on creating a safe environment, aiming at symptom management and self-care.
9. Family doctors should deliver proactive care, with one coordinating care provider, and a stepped-care approach.
10. Family doctors should develop "cultural competence".

# Definition of MUS

Medically unexplained symptoms (MUS) are physical symptoms that have existed for several weeks and for which adequate medical examination or investigation have not revealed any condition that sufficiently explains the symptoms.

Physical symptoms such as headaches, back pain, chest pain, abdominal pain, dizziness and feelings of weakness or fatigue are common. Two-thirds of men and four-fifths of women say they have had at least one physical symptom in the last two weeks. Only a minority visit the doctor with these symptoms. In a quarter to a half of these symptoms, the family doctor is unable to diagnose an underlying disease. In 80% of the cases, one visit to the family doctor is enough and the symptoms will resolve.

**Table 4.1** Functional syndromes in specialty care

| Speciality | Syndromes |
|---|---|
| Gynaecology | Chronic pelvic pain, premenstrual syndrome |
| Gastroenterology | Irritable bowel syndrome, non-ulcer dyspepsia |
| Neurology | Tension headache, non-epileptic seizures |
| Internal medicine | Chronic fatigue syndrome/myalgic encephalomyelitis |
| Cardiology | Atypical chest pain, benign palpitations |
| Rheumatology | Fibromyalgia |
| Orthopaedics | Low back pain, repetitive strain injury |
| Ear, nose, throat | Idiopathic tinnitus, globus syndrome |
| Respiratory | Hyperventilation syndrome |

Up to 40% of the consultations in primary care concern symptoms for which no adequate somatic condition can be found. The prevalence of persistent severe MUS is approximately 2.5%.

Medical specialties tend to classify MUS into functional somatic syndromes. However, these functional syndromes overlap in their symptoms, aetiology and treatments. Table 4.1 lists the most common functional somatic syndromes by specialty.[1]

MUS is a working hypothesis based on the (justified) assumption that somatic or psychiatric pathology have been adequately detected and treated but the clinical condition presented by the patient was not adequately resolved. Any change in symptoms could be a reason to revise the working hypothesis of MUS.[2]

For some patients with physical symptoms a somatic or psychiatric condition may be present, but if the physical symptoms are more severe or more persistent or limit functioning to a greater extent than expected based on the condition in question, they too are referred to as MUS.

MUS can be seen as a continuum ranging from self-limiting symptoms, to recurrent and/or persisting symptoms and symptom disorders.

# Causes of MUS

In 1977 George Engel introduced the biopsychosocial model. This model implies that in order to give patients a sense of being understood, clinicians have to understand and respond adequately to patients' suffering. In order to achieve this, clinicians must attend simultaneously to the biological, psychological and social dimensions of illness. This biopsychosocial model is fully integrated in the philosophy of primary care.

The term MUS implies there is no clear explanation for the origin of the symptoms. However, factors that play a role in MUS can be categorized into predisposing, precipitating (i.e. exacerbating) and perpetuating (i.e. maintaining) factors. These factors can be linked to the biopsychosocial model, as we set out in Table 4.2. The different elements of the biopsychosocial model and the predisposing, precipitating and perpetuating factors can play a role in

**Table 4.2** Predisposing, precipitating, perpetuating factors, and the biopsychosocial model in MUS

**Predisposing factors**

| Biological | Psychological | Social |
|---|---|---|
| Genetics | Current life stresses | Illness experience in family |
| Chronic health problems | Psychological trauma | Illness behavior in family |
| Serious childhood illness | Adverse childhood experiences | Neglecting self-care of personal needs |
| | Physical, sexual or emotional abuse (in childhood) | Cultural beliefs and expectations |
| | Unsafe parental bonding | Health systems characteristics |
| | Depression | |
| | Anxiety disorders | |
| | Post-traumatic stress | |
| | Other psychiatric disorders | |
| | Personality characteristics (alexithymia, neuroticism) | |

**Precipitating factors**

| | | |
|---|---|---|
| Decrease ability to exercise | Inability to modify current worries and anxiety | Lack of social support |
| Decreased capacity and resilience | Depression | Illness gain |
| Increased sensitivity and perception (sensitization, hypervigiliance) | Dysfunctional illness cognitions | Learned behavior |
| | Low self-esteem | Family dynamics |
| | False attributions | |
| | Catastrophizing thoughts | |
| | Role and behavior of the clinician | |

| Infectious diseases | Stress overload | Negative life-events (loss of |
|---|---|---|
| Accident/trauma | Depression | a beloved one, impending |
| Surgery | Anxiety disorders | resignation) |
| | Other psychiatric | Difficult living conditions |
| | disorders | High workload |
| | Recent life event | Limited social support on |
| | linked to past trauma | work |
| | Ongoing contact with | Mass media reports on |
| | abusive important | health issues/concerns |
| | others | |

**Perpetuating factors**

| Decrease ability to exercise | Inability to modify cur- | Lack of social support |
|---|---|---|
| Decreased capacity and | rent worries and | Illness gain |
| resilience | anxiety | Learned behavior |
| Increased sensitivity and | Depression | Family dynamics |
| perception (sensitization, | Dysfunctional illness | |
| hypervigiliance) | cognitions | |
| | Low self-esteem | |
| | False attributions | |
| | Catastrophizing | |
| | thoughts | |
| | Role and behavior of | |
| | the clinician | |

varying degrees in understanding the causes of MUS. Furthermore, they can be used in the explanation of MUS during the clinical encounter.

# Diagnosing MUS

MUS always remains a working hypothesis, as in a limited number of cases it could become clear over time that the symptoms were in fact caused by somatic pathology.[3] In the case of alarming symptoms (according to the family doctor) or changes in the pattern of symptoms (according to the patient), the working hypothesis MUS should be reconsidered and physical re-examination or additional investigations might be needed.[2]

### Exploration of symptoms
The biopsychosocial model proposes illness to be viewed as a result of interacting mechanisms at the biomedical, interpersonal and environmental or contextual levels. Therefore the exploration of symptoms in patients with MUS should focus on the exact chronology of the symptoms themselves, including where and when the symptoms appear (context of the symptoms);

which potential causes of MUS are present, patients' ideas, concerns and expectations (i.e. ICE); patients' illness behavior, the patient's life and the social environment of the patient.

This exploration results in a better understanding of the patient and the nature of the symptoms.[4]

Here is a list of symptom dimensions, with sample questions:

1. **Symptom focus**. "Which specific symptoms are bothering you at the moment?" (Location, duration, severity, pattern, accompanying symptoms, use of medication).
2. **Ideas**. "What are your own ideas and thoughts about these symptoms?" (Origin and persistence of the symptoms (including chronological aspects and when symptoms are present), contributing factors to the symptoms, patient's own influence on the symptoms, what aspects of their lives the patients considered to be associated with the symptoms).
3. **Concerns**. "Do you have any concerns or worries about these symptoms?" (Anxiety or panic for what exactly, uncertainty, depressed, despair).
4. **Effects**. "What effect do these symptoms have on you?" (Absence of work, avoidance of physical activity, ignoring the symptoms, other behaviors that inhibit recovery). "Do these symptoms interfere with your daily life and social activities?"
5. **Reaction of others**. "How do other people react to your symptoms?" (Relationships, friendships, work).
6. **Expectations**. "What do you expect will happen with your symptoms in the future?" "What do you expect from treatments for your symptoms?"

### Exploration of potential psychosocial contributing factors

As MUS can often (but not always) be linked to psychosocial stress, the family doctor needs to pay attention to these issues. Important in this regard is to listen very carefully to what patients communicate. In 95% of the MUS consultations patients present psychosocial cues or hints. However, it is important that family doctors do not ignore these cues. Picking up these cues and exploring them in depth by using open ended questions ("What do you mean by [ ... ]?") often results in a deeper understanding of the patient's symptoms. When psychosocial stress is present, discussing and treating these issues often leads to symptomatic improvement.

Here is a list of these psychosocial problems, with sample questions:

1. **Current life stresses**. "Are you experiencing stress at the moment?" "Did you have a stressful experience just before the start of your symptoms?"
2. **Limited self-care skills**. "Do you care for others but have difficulty putting yourself on the list of people for whom you care?"
3. **Adverse childhood experiences (ACEs)**. "Were you under stress as a child?" "Would you feel sad or angry if a child you care about was growing up just as you did?" "Do you still interact with anyone who mistreated you as a child?"
4. **High workload**. "What work do you do at the moment?" "Do you like your job?" "How are your working hours?" "Do you take work home with you?"
5. **Problems in interpersonal relationships**. "Do you face problems in relationships with important others?"

### Identifying comorbid psychiatric disorders

As patients with anxiety disorder, depression or post traumatic stress disorder (PTSD) can present with physical symptoms, for example, fatigue or palpitations, it is important to explore whether there is a comorbid anxiety disorder, depression or PTSD (see also above). Furthermore, the presence of a comorbid psychiatric disorder can be a predisposing or precipitating factor in MUS. In case such a comorbid psychiatric disorder is present the clinician must first treat the comorbid psychiatric disorder according to the existing guidelines (see, for example, the WHO "mhGAP intervention guide 2.0"). For diagnosing and treating anxiety disorder, depression or PTSD we refer to existing disease specific guidelines. When this treatment proceeds, the working hypothesis MUS can be reconsidered based on the remaining symptoms.

### Evaluation

Based on the exploration of symptoms (and with it the identification of predisposing, precipitating and perpetuating factors), the clinician is able to evaluate the severity of MUS. MUS can be considered on a severity scale from mild via moderate to severe. The greater the number and the longer the duration of symptoms presented, the more number of bodily systems affected (for example, gastrointestinal, cardiopulmonary, musculoskeletal), the more number of consultations with physicians and the more the level of functioning is impaired, the greater the severity of MUS is. The severity established by the physician guides the stepped-care approach described below.[2]

# Managing MUS

We distinguish a number of important elements in the management of MUS. Most of these elements and their content are described in and extracted from a recent review of national guidelines and Cochrane reviews.[4]

### Importance of the doctor–patient relationship

Patients with MUS evoke difficulties in the family doctor encounter and challenge the doctor–patient relationship. A good doctor–patient relationship is associated with patient satisfaction and improved health outcomes and is an important condition for a good treatment course. Furthermore, the doctor–patient relationship can be strengthened by recognizing the patient's illness, taking the patient and his/her symptoms seriously, and showing empathy and interest in the patient's life context and problems that are related to the presence of MUS. The family doctor should take an open, empathic, active supporting attitude to the symptoms and their management, in order to build a sustainable and equal working relationship. The physician needs to convey to the patient that the impact of the symptoms is understood and the physician acts with sensitivity to the difficulties that the patient experiences. The management of patients with MUS is most successful when there is a continuing and warm doctor–patient relationship.[4]

### Importance of doctor–patient communication

Doctor–patient communication is essential for the treatment of MUS, as patients seek understanding of their symptoms. To achieve this, the family doctor should focus on their consultation skills:

1. A structured exploration of the symptoms;
2. Pay attention to cues and hints;
3. Provide a summary;
4. Explicit communication about expected results of biomedical investigations.

So, family doctors should explore the patient's reasons for encounter, ideas, concerns and expectations (ICE) about the symptoms, and assess for potential predisposing, precipitating and perpetuating in a structured way using open questions. This exploration validates the patient's sense of suffering and provides a detailed insight into the biopsychosocial background of the symptoms which is needed for a shared understanding of the symptoms. Paying attention to cues and hints in the story of the patients (i.e. the psychosocial background of the symptoms) can be reached by listening attentively and very carefully to what the patient is telling you and by asking open questions in order to reach an understanding of the cues and hints provided. Provision of a summary by the family doctor is a tool in the communication with these patients. Such a summary should include the topics that have been discussed in the consultation. It gives the patient the opportunity to check whether the doctor understands the problem and to complement deficits. Explicit communication about expected results of biomedical investigations is essential. When discussing treatment, the doctor should communicate with the patient in an open and accommodating dialogue in which the advantages and disadvantages of further testing and treatment can be discussed.[4]

## Importance of explanation

Family doctors should provide a targeted and tangible explanation in the patient's language and cultural models about what is causing the symptoms. Information obtained during the structured exploration of the symptoms should be incorporated in this explanation. Patients benefit from an "explanation that makes sense, removes any blame from the patient, and generates ideas about how to manage the symptoms."[5] Recent research on explanations provides suggestions for constructing plausible and acceptable explanations for symptoms. Patients need to be able to exchange ideas with their doctors on the explanatory models they have and build up a common understanding on how these symptoms develop within explanatory models that are culturally acceptable, especially when the biological links between problems, emotions and symptoms are clarified.

Explanations that are cocreated by the patient and the family doctor are most likely to be accepted by the patient.[6] However, although evidence for the effectiveness of those explanatory models in reassuring patients is limited, a patient-centred approach is always the best model to improve self-management and patient empowerment. According to existing consensus, targeted and tangible explanations in the patient's language and cultural models are necessary to reassure patients with MUS about the absence of a somatic disease.

One general explanation that most patients can comprehend is that when a person's stress level is too high or persists for too long, this can lead to physical symptoms very much like tension can lead to headache, fearful situations can cause a "knot" in the abdomen or embarrassment can cause blushing.

Here are some examples of explanatory models that can be used in daily primary care:[2]

1. **Capacity–burden model:**
   The balance between four factors (i.e. support, stress, strength and vulnerability) is of importance. If vulnerability and strength are unbalanced in a person, this can lead to symptoms.

2. **Stress model:**
   High levels of stress are correlated with fatigue, pain and somatoform disorders. Psychological distress plays an important role in this relationship. That means that certain psychosocial factors combined with a chronically high level of stress can result in MUS.

3. **Somatosensory amplification model:**
   Focusing attention on physical sensations leads to more physical sensations (for example, thinking of itching results in itching). Furthermore, this might result in concerns or anxiety in patients. Consequently, a vicious circle of maintaining and amplifying the physical symptoms is started.

4. **Neurobiological model:**
   There exists a complex interaction between neurobiological processes (the autonomic nervous system, the HPA axis and the immune system), environmental factors, attention and behavior. Activation of the autonomic nervous systems generates symptoms, as does activation of the HPA axis (for example, adrenalin gives an increase in heartrate and breathing frequency). Activation of the immune system can result in a sickness response.

5. **Vicious circles:**
   Vicious circles play an important role in maintaining symptoms, irrespective of the origin of the symptoms. This is a result of the interpretation of symptoms and resulting disease behavior and/or help-seeking behavior.

6. **Sensitization:**
   Previous and repeated stimuli of pain and other symptoms in the past make the central nervous system more susceptible to these stimuli. Benign stimuli are interpreted as malign.

7. **Cultural way of understanding:**
   All explanatory models must be culturally meaningful. It is important for health professionals to be culturally humble, respecting and

understanding of how different cultures explain the many ways emotional distress relates to physical symptoms. One example is the "nerves" complaints among Latino patients that associate "shaken nerves" as a major mechanism causing MUS.

## Symptom management

Many patients with MUS improve without specific treatment. Although around 30% of the symptoms that patients present to their family doctor are unexplained (in specialist care this is even higher, up to 70%) only a minority of these MUS become persistent and disabling.[7]

When symptoms persist for more than several weeks, the physician may decide to prescribe medications addressing the specific symptom(s) presented, for example, analgesics for pain, tricyclic antidepressants for neuropathic pain, or beta blockers for disturbing tachycardia. This symptom management aiming at symptomatic relief via physiological means is advisable especially in the initial phase. When considering pain management, short term analgesia with, for example, acetaminophen or a non steroid anti inflammatory drug (NSAID) (if no contraindication) can be prescribed. In all cases family doctors have to balance symptomatic treatment with potential adverse effects or risks.[8]

A Cochrane review on pharmacological treatments for patients with MUS concluded that there is little evidence for the effectiveness of medication (tricyclic antidepressants), new-generation antidepressants (i.e. SSRIs and SNRIs) and natural products (i.e. different herbs and St. John's wort) in the treatment of patients with MUS.[9]

## Self-care and self-management

The physician can advise patients on self-management strategies and self-care. The physician can empower the patient to carry on with (or return to) their normal daily activities as much as possible despite experiencing symptoms. The physician can suggest scheduling activities and exercises, practicing a regular sleep pattern, practicing a regular and healthy diet and relaxation exercises.[10,11]

Self-help and behavioral activation can reduce symptoms and improve quality of life of patients with MUS. Engagement in pleasurable activities such as regular exercise, pursuit of a hobby or social activities can counteract the discomfort or suffering from MUS and reduce stress. We have discussed these options in more detail in Chapter 3.

**A stepped-care approach**

Family doctors should deliver proactive care and make regular follow-up appointments during the course of treatment based on the patient's need. Furthermore, it is important that one care provider, preferably the family doctor, keeps control and coordination of the care process. However, this care provider could also be a community psychiatric nurse, psychologist or occupational health physician.

The stages of severity of the symptoms can be connected to management options in a stepped-care approach. Family doctors should assess the patient's risk profile on the basis of the severity of the MUS and the complexity of the disorder (number and duration of symptoms, level of functional impairment, psychosocial stress, psychological comorbidity and experienced difficulties in the doctor–patient relationship). Table 4.3 shows the stepped-care approach, as described in several primary care guidelines.

The more severe or complex the symptoms and limitations are, the more intense and complex is the treatment needed for the recovery of the patient. For example, when stress has been uncovered during the exploration of the symptoms of a patient with mild MUS, stress relief is often the only treatment needed to relieve MUS.

This can be done by:

1. Asking patients to compile a list of significant life stresses both present and past and searching together on how to reduce one or more stresses;
2. Recommending 2 to 5 hours of self-care time (purely for personal enjoyment) every week; and/or
3. Suggesting relaxation techniques and/or mindfulness meditation.

In patients with moderate to severe MUS, referral to mental healthcare could be indicated. The most severely affected patients need a close collaboration between professionals with a divergent range of skills and expertise in secondary or tertiary care (i.e. the final step in the stepped-care approach).

# Cultural issues in managing MUS

Physical symptoms are an important part of different "idioms of distress", which are socially accepted patterns of presenting emotional distress (including anxiety and depressive disorders) that vary due to cultural background. There are several factors that contribute to these patterns, including

**Table 4.3** Stepped-care approach to managing MUS

| | Dutch family doctor guideline | Danish family doctor guideline | German multidisciplinary guideline | Dutch multidisciplinary guideline |
|---|---|---|---|---|
| **Mild MUS** | - Psychoeducation<br>- (Self-)management advice<br>- Shared time-contingent plan<br>- Follow-up | **Symptoms and mild functional disorders**<br>- Normalization, explanation, biopsychosocial approach<br>- Follow-up | **Step 1**<br>- General principles of therapy (empathy, watchful waiting, acknowledgement of the symptoms, explanation)<br>- Therapy by family doctor or medical specialist or psychosomatic primary health care | **Mild MUS**<br>- Biopsychosocial approach by family doctor<br>- Psychoeducation<br>- Short-term CBT |
| **Moderate MUS** | - Psychosomatic physio/exercise therapy<br>- Mental health nurse practitioner<br>- Social psychiatric nurse | **Moderate functional disorders**<br>- Explanations and TERM model[a]<br>- Regular consultations<br>- Cooperation with specialist (in charge of assessment, treatment plan and supervision) | **Step 2**<br>- Regular consultations<br>- Therapy by family doctor or medical specialist PLUS psychotherapy<br>- Pain as core symptom: antidepressant<br>- Pain not as core symptom: antidepressant in case of psychiatric comorbidity | **Moderate MUS**<br>- Case management by medical specialist, psychiatrist or family doctor<br>- Medication (for comorbidity)<br>- CBT |

Table 4.3 (Cont.)

| Dutch family doctor guideline | Danish family doctor guideline | German multidisciplinary guideline | Dutch multidisciplinary guideline |
|---|---|---|---|
| **Severe MUS** | **Severe functional disorders** | **Step 3** | **Severe MUS** |
| - Multidisciplinary team/treatment centre | - Specialist clinic<br>- Multidisciplinary treatment<br>- CBT[b] and GET[c]<br>- Consider pharmacological treatment | - Specialist clinic with multidisciplinary treatment | - CBT<br>- Treatment by a multidisciplinary team in tertiary care |

Source: adapted from olde Hartman et al. 2017
Notes:
a. The Extended Reattribution and Management model
b. Cognitive behavioral therapy
c. Graded exercise therapy

some previously discussed in this chapter, but the culturally accepted way to communicate and elaborate on emotional suffering is one of the core points, especially when "individualist" or "collectivist" cultures are involved. In the former, personal and subjective ways of expressing emotional distress are valued, while in the latter preserving group cohesion is the most important point and so it is considered inadequate to verbalize feelings and emotions associated with conflicts or negative emotions. But the physical symptoms associated with emotional distress cannot be suppressed, may become quite disturbing and disabling, and represent the most important reason for searching health care.

Trying to build an international cultural background when MUS are concerned may be quite difficult. On the one hand, it has been found that the most frequent groups of physical symptoms associated with MUS, currently being studied as "Bodily Stress Syndrome", are universal and similar to those found in previously described "cultural-bound syndromes", such as "Hwa-Byung" in Korea or as "Nervios" in Latin America. On the other hand, functional syndromes are not acknowledged and diagnosed in the same way worldwide. Recognition of chronic fatigue syndrome in Brazil and UK differ dramatically within a similar frequency of core symptoms in the general population of the two countries.[12]

The most important consequence of this problem is the need for primary care physicians to develop cultural competence when dealing with migrants or culturally heterogeneous populations. The "Cultural Formulation Interview"[13] can be used to help professionals approach patients from different backgrounds. It recognizes the importance of cultural determinants in everyday practice in health care.[14,15] We discuss this further in Chapter 6, when considering the mental health of migrants.

## Service delivery

Every family doctor encounters patients with MUS. Good consultation and communications skills and building a therapeutic relationship with these patients are prerequisites in high quality management of MUS. Furthermore, collaboration with the patient and with other health care professionals in primary, secondary and mental health care is essential. Most patients with MUS don't have to be treated in secondary care as family doctors are in the good position to deliver patients with MUS the high quality of care they need. It is important that one care provider, preferably the family doctor, keeps control and coordination of the care process. However, this care provider could also be a community psychiatric nurse, psychologist or occupational health physician. Furthermore, it should be clear to the patient with MUS which care provider keeps control and coordination of the care process.

# Educational material

## Case study

A 31-year-old woman consults you for the third time because she has persistent fatigue and pain in her muscles. She is worried because she is not able to work and not able to take care of her family. The fatigue is persistent, and the pain in the muscles gets worse during the day. By the end of the day she has to lie in her bed or on the sofa and she is not able to do her normal daily activities.

Physical examination and special investigations, including blood tests and the consultation of a rheumatologist, did not reveal any abnormalities.

*What should you do next?*
- Explore the symptoms in depth.
- Identify comorbid psychiatric disorders.
- Provide the patient with an explanation that everything is normal.

At this stage it is important to explore the patient's symptoms in depth. Using the standard consultation technique of ICE (ideas, concerns and expectations) you ask your patient what she thinks might be causing her fatigue and pain in her muscles. Furthermore, you ask how much she worries about her symptoms. You ask her how you can help her with her symptoms.

She tells you that she wants to know why she has the fatigue and the pain. When you tell her that often fatigue and pain is nothing to worry about, she gets angry and tells about her neighbor who had the same symptoms and ultimately got cancer.

You listen and react empathically and tell her that you understand her anxiety. Furthermore, you explain to her that you know that she is suffering from real fatigue and real pain, and that you will try to help her with that.

When you ask her about her work, she gets emotional and tells you that there is too much work and that she has had arguments with her boss. It all started when her boss came back from sick leave.

*What do you tell her?*
- That she has an anxiety disorder.
- That you are not able to take her fatigue and pain away because she doesn't have a disease, it seems to be stress, so she should visit a psychologist.
- You explain that the tests you have already done show that she does not have cancer, and that she is generally in good physical health.

It is valuable to inform her that she does not have a serious disease such as cancer. You know that fatigue and pain are commonly presented symptoms in primary care and that when thorough (additional) investigation does not reveal any abnormalities that most of these symptoms stay unexplained. You are aware that such symptoms can originate from stressful life events or psychosocial stress. Given the problems of her work you consider that this might be a perpetuating factor of the symptoms. Furthermore you recognize her emotions regarding the cancer of her neighbor.

*What explanation do you give her?*
- That there doesn't seem to be a problem with her general health and muscles as the rheumatologist and the blood tests revealed nothing serious.
- That her fatigue and muscle pain involve multiple factors. The situation of her neighbor might have triggered her symptoms. The problems with her work can perpetuate her symptoms. Stress takes up a lot of energy and when energy is already low than a person can run out of energy, resulting in fatigue.
- You don't give an explanation to her as her symptoms are medically unexplained. This means that an explanation is not possible.

It is helpful to provide an explanation for symptoms which is grounded in the patient's own ideas and concerns. Therefore we recommend the second of these choices.

She realizes that the stress from her work is the most important problem right now. She agrees that her sleeping pattern is affected as she experiences a lot of tension when she is lying in her bed. She asks what to do about this.

Tim olde Hartman et al.

*What is an appropriate management plan?*
- You prescribe an antidepressant or tranquiliser.
- You send her to a multidisciplinary treatment team.
- You propose behavioral activation, relaxation exercises, help her to identify and involve supportive family and friends and ask her to make a new appointment at your consultation hour in two weeks.

There are many things that you can do to help your patient manage her problems more effectively. We therefore recommend the third of these choices. You can read more about these useful techniques in Chapter 3.

# Multiple choice questions

1. Which of the following statements is correct?

   a. MUS are psychological symptoms that have existed for several months and for which adequate medical examination or investigation have not revealed any medical condition that sufficiently explains the symptoms.
   b. MUS are psychological symptoms that have existed for several weeks and for which adequate medical examination or investigation have not revealed any medical condition that sufficiently explains the symptoms.
   c. MUS is a diagnosis, based on the (justified) assumption that somatic or psychiatric pathology have been adequately detected and treated but the clinical condition presented by the patient was not adequately resolved.
   d. MUS is a working hypothesis, based on the (justified) assumption that somatic or psychiatric pathology have been adequately detected and treated but the clinical condition presented by the patient was not adequately resolved.

2. Which of the following is a perpetuating factor of MUS?

   a. Adverse childhood experiences.
   b. Worries and anxiety.
   c. Infectious diseases.
   d. Limited social support.

3. Which is the correct order to reach the working hypothesis MUS? (1: Exploration of symptoms; 2: Evaluation of severity of MUS; 3: Identifying comorbid psychiatric disorders; 4: Exploration of potential psychosocial contributing factors)

   a. 2 – 1 – 3 – 4
   b. 3 – 4 – 1 – 2
   c. 1 – 3 – 4 – 2
   d. 1 – 4 – 3 – 2

4. Which of the following elements in the management of MUS is considered least important?

   a. Drug treatment.
   b. Building a therapeutic doctor–patient relationship.
   c. Providing a targeted and tangible explanation.
   d. Genuine doctor–patient communication.

5. What is the correct order of a stepped-care approach (from mild to moderate to severe) in MUS? (1: psychoeducation; 2: referral to a multidisciplinary team; 3: referral to psychotherapist; 4: regular consultations)

   a. 1 – 2 – 3 – 4
   b. 1 – 4 – 3 – 2
   c. 4 – 3 – 1 – 2
   d. 4 – 1 – 2 – 3

You will find the answers to these MCQs on page 171.

# References

1. Sharpe M. Medically unexplained symptoms and syndromes. *Clin Med* 2002, 2(6):501–504.
2. Olde Hartman TC, Blankenstein AH, Molenaar B, et al. NHG Standaard SOLK [NHG Guideline on Medically Unexplained Symptoms (MUS)]. *Huisarts en Wetenschap* 2013, 56(5):222. (www.nhg.org/sites/default/files/content/nhg_org/uploads/standaard/download/final_m102_solk_guideline_sk_mei13_0.pdf).
3. Morriss R, Dowrick C, Salmon P, et al. Cluster randomised controlled trial of training practices in reattribution for medically unexplained symptoms. *Br J Psychiatr* 2007, 191:536–542.
4. Olde Hartman TC, Rosendal M, Aamland A, et al. What do guidelines and systematic reviews tell us about the management of medically unexplained symptoms in primary care? *BJGP Open* 2017. doi: 10.3399/bjgpopen17X101061.

5. Burton C, Lucassen P, Aamland A, et al. Explaining symptoms after negative tests: towards a rational explanation. *J R Soc Med* 2015, 108(3):84–88.
6. Den Boeft M, Huisman D, Morton L, et al. Negotiating explanations: doctor-patient communication with patients with medically unexplained symptoms – a qualitative analysis. *Fam Pract* 2017, 34(1):107–113.
7. Verhaak PFM, Meijer SA, Visser AP, et al. Persistent presentation of medically unexplained symptoms in general practice. *Fam Pract* 2006, 23(4):414–420.
8. Chitnis A, Dowrick C, Byng R, et al. *Guidance for health professionals on medically unexplained symptoms.* London: Royal College of General Practitioners and Royal College of Psychiatrists, 2014.
9. Kleinstauber M, Witthoft M, Steffanowski A, et al. Pharmacological interventions for somatoform disorders in adults. *Cochrane Database Syst Rev* 2014, 7(11):CD010628.
10. Van Gils A, Schoevers RA, Bonvanie IJ, et al. Self-help for medically unexplained symptoms: a systematic review and meta-analysis. *Psychosom Med* 2016, 78 (6):728–739.
11. Henningsen P, Zipfel S, Herzog W. Management of functional somatic syndromes. *Lancet* 2007, 369:946–955.
12. Cho HJ, Menezes PR, Bhugra D, et al. The awareness of chronic fatigue syndrome: a comparative study in Brazil and the United Kingdom. *J Psychsom Res* 2008, 64 (4):351–355.
13. DSM5 cultural formulation interview. www.psychiatry.org/File%20Library/Psychiatrists/ Practice/DSM/APA_DSM5_Cultural-Formulation-Interview.pdf
14. Kirmayer L, Ban L. Cultural psychiatry: research strategies and future directions. *Adv Psychosom Med* 2013, 33:97–114.
15. Lewis-Fernandez RL, Kirmayer LJ, Garnaccia P, et al. Cultural concepts of distress, in Sadock B, Sadock V, Ruiz P. (Eds). *Comprehensive textbook of psychiatry.* New York: Lippincott, Williams and Wilkins, 2017.

Chapter 5

# PHYSICAL HEALTH CARE OF PEOPLE WITH SEVERE MENTAL ILLNESS

Alan Cohen and Kim Griswold

# Key points

1. The Family Doctor (FD) and his or her team should approach the management of the physical health of people with a severe mental illness (SMI) in the same way as for any other long-term condition.
2. If there are registers of people with diabetes, cardiovascular disease, or other non-communicable diseases (NCD) then there should be a register of people with an SMI.
3. If the FD manages NCD by opportunistic screening in the general population, then NCD should be screened opportunistically in the SMI population.
4. Every patient should have their BP and BMI (body mass index) recorded in the clinical record, at least annually.
5. If the FD usually manages NCD in the general population, then the FD should assess people with SMI for the development of those NCD and manage them in the same way as they would for people without an SMI.
6. If the FD does not usually manage specific NCD, then the FD should arrange for people with SMI to be assessed by clinicians who are able to manage these conditions.
7. If the FD normally enquires about smoking habits, then the patient should be assessed, and if appropriate, offered smoking cessation advice. Their respiratory function should be assessed and appropriate treatment offered.
8. Preventative strategies offered to at risk groups should be offered to people with SMI, e.g. influenza vaccination, screening for bowel cancer, screening for cervical cancer, screening for BBV (blood borne viral) disorders etc., if these programmes exist, and are applied routinely for other patients.
9. Management:
   a. Where clinically indicated, lifestyle changes should be offered as a first-line in the management of NCD.
   b. If lifestyle changes are inappropriate, or ineffective, for an individual then medication should be offered in line with national guidelines and best practice.
   c. The FD will need to balance the benefits of more medication to treat/prevent a potentially life-shortening condition, and the risks associated with polypharmacy.

  d. In assessing the "risk versus benefit" the FD should take into account:

   i The views and opinions of the patient;
   ii The cultural context of the patient and family;
   iii The lifestyle and social circumstances of the patient;
   iv The clinical evidence that supports the proposed intervention;
   v The risk of drug interactions.

  e. The FD should assess each patient's beliefs and preferences and assess levels of health literacy and barriers to care.
  f. The FD should use interpreters as appropriate for patients with language barriers.
  g. Patients should be provided with self-management support from lay health coaches, navigators, or community health workers when available.

# Introduction

Individuals with severe mental illness (SMI) suffer a disproportionate burden of non-communicable diseases (NCD) and can expect a life span 25 years shorter than the general population.[1] Millennium Sustainable Goal 3 aims "to reduce premature mortality from non-communicable diseases (NCD) through prevention and treatment and promote mental health and well-being"; a goal that is imperative for people with severe mental illness.[2,3]

### Definition of SMI

The term "severe mental illness" is frequently used but is imprecise in its nature. In the generally accepted form, the term has three elements: Diagnosis, Disability and Duration.

- **Diagnosis:** A diagnosis of schizophrenia, bipolar disorder, or other psychotic disorder is usually implied.
- **Disability:** The disorder causes significant disability.
- **Duration:** The disorder has lasted for a significant duration, usually at least two years.

Family doctors are in an ideal position to recognise, and/or treat or refer patients they see in general care. This chapter will present an evidence-based approach to management of patients with SMI emphasising the treatment of non-communicable diseases.

# Type 2 diabetes in people with a severe mental illness

### What is the prevalence of diabetes in people with SMI?

The prevalence rate for diabetes amongst people with severe mental illness is around two to three times that found in the general population.[4,5] The causes of the increased prevalence are probably multifactorial and include genetic causes, social causes and iatrogenic causes. It is interesting to note that Sir Henry Maudsley in the 1890s, before the invention of antipsychotic medication, had identified that diabetes was more common amongst people with dementia praecox, as schizophrenia was then known.

### What are the risk factors for people with SMI?

There are a number of risk factors for diabetes for people with SMI. People with SMI are more likely to be overweight, and more likely to lead a sedentary lifestyle. They are more likely to have poor nutrition, which is linked with the increase in social deprivation that is characteristic of these disorders. They are more likely to be prescribed antipsychotic medication, and are more likely to have dyslipidaemia. They are more likely to lead a chaotic lifestyle, which in itself makes access to primary and preventative care more complicated.

### What are the effects of anti-psychotic medication?

Second generation anti-psychotic medication is recognised to induce the metabolic syndrome, of which Type 2 diabetes is part. Studies show that it is the medication that plays a significant role in the development of the metabolic syndrome, rather than the illness for which the medication is prescribed. All anti-psychotic medication has the potential to unmask or cause Type 2 diabetes.[6]

### What is the effect of lifestyle choices and social determinants of health?

People with severe mental illness access health care services less than others, and therefore do not take up offers of diabetes prevention as frequently as others. They are more likely to be unemployed, and homeless, and therefore less able to afford medication that might be prescribed for the treatment of diabetes.

### What is the effect of multi-morbidity?

People with severe mental illness are more likely to have a metabolic syndrome, which includes diabetes. Diabetes is itself a risk factor for cardiovascular disease, and the complications of diabetes such as renal failure and erectile dysfunction are independent risk factors for cardiovascular disease.

### What are the recommendations for clinical care?

- Annually screen people who are prescribed atypical anti-psychotic medications for prediabetes or diabetes.
- The diagnosis of diabetes should be made using fasting blood glucose levels, using the current WHO definition of diabetes and prediabetes. HbA1c should not be used to diagnose diabetes. This is because the blood glucose level can rise very quickly when anti-psychotic medication is prescribed, much more quickly than the 90-day life-span of erythrocytes on which the HbA1c measurement is based.
- Dyslipidaemia should be assessed annually. The diagnosis and management of dyslipidaemia should be based on national or regional guidelines.
- A HbA1c should be performed quarterly in individuals whose glycemic control is not optimum. As part of treatment planning, a target HbA1c should be agreed with each person that reflects individual circumstances and current medical history. The target should be reviewed annually as part of the routine diabetic review.
- The monitoring of diabetes self-care activities should be incorporated into the treatment goals in people with diabetes and severe mental illness.[7]

# Smoking and respiratory disease in people with a severe mental illness

### What is the prevalence in people with SMI?

One in three of all cigarettes smoked are smoked by people with a mental health condition. In the general population, smoking has fallen by 25% in the last two decades, although there has not been a similar decline in smoking amongst people with a mental health condition. Smoking is more prevalent amongst people with mental health disorders, e.g. 45% of people with schizophrenia who live in the community smoke cigarettes, and this figure rises to 80% for those living in long term residential facilities.[8] The groups most likely to smoke are the young (16–25), those with long standing mental health problems, e.g. schizophrenia, and those who come from lower socio-economic groupings. People with a long term mental health problem may wish to quit smoking, but are more likely to expect to fail, compared to the general population. Smoking cessation interventions that utilise the principles of motivational interviewing are effective in this group, as well as some medication, e.g. varenicline.[9]

### What are the effects of anti-psychotic medication?

There is an important interaction between cigarette smoking and anti-psychotic medication. Cigarette smoking increases the metabolism of some anti-psychotic medication so that to achieve the same drug response, a higher dose of medication is needed in smokers. The evidence for clozapine demonstrates that a reduction of up to 25% of the dose is required when a patient stops smoking. Leaving the dose unchanged when a patient stops smoking tobacco risks the patient suffering toxic levels of the medication.[10]

### What are the effects of lifestyle choices and social determinants of health?

There is strong evidence that programmes tailored specifically for the needs of SMI are effective in achieving smoking cessation. Acceptance rates for these programmes are similar to programmes designed for the general population and outcomes are similar to programmes designed for the general population.[11] Medication such as varenicline used in smoking cessation programmes is safe for people with SMI. The major difference between the SMI group and the general population is that the former have a higher expectation of failure.

### What is the effect of multi-morbidity?

The commonest cause of death amongst people with SMI is pneumonia. 40% of all cases of chronic respiratory disease are caused by smoking and so it is not a surprise that chronic obstructive pulmonary disease is more common amongst people with SMI. Rates vary around the world, but it is 2 to 3 times more common for people with SMI living in the community, and for institutions where up to 80% of in-patients smoke, very much greater.[12] Smoking will exacerbate the management of diabetes, the management of cardiovascular disease, and increase the risk of thrombosis – all of which are more common in people with SMI. Anti-psychotic medication is also thrombophilic. After deprivation and smoking are factored into the statistics, lung cancer is not more common in people with SMI. However proportionately lung cancer is more common because a greater proportion of people with SMI smoke, and as they present later for diagnosis and treatment, it is more likely to be fatal.[13]

**What are the recommendations for clinical care?**
- In all countries, every person with SMI should be asked on an annual basis if they smoke tobacco. The response should be recorded in the clinical record.
- In every country smoking cessation advice should be offered to people with SMI who do smoke tobacco. Advice that is effective utilises the principles of motivational interviewing.
- For those people with SMI who do smoke tobacco, they should be offered simple spirometry investigations to assess if they are developing chronic respiratory diseases such as chronic obstructive pulmonary disease. Where chronic respiratory conditions are developing, early treatment and advice should be offered, and these people should be followed up in the same way that others in the general population are followed and regularly reviewed.
- Mental health hospitals should ban smoking for in-patients and staff.

# Cardiovascular disease in people with a severe mental illness

### What is the prevalence of the disorder in people with SMI?
Causes of death amongst people with schizophrenia from cardiovascular disease increased from 1.84 times greater than the general population in the 1970s, to over 3.20 times greater in the 1990s. This increase has continued into the 21st century, whilst the equivalent rate for people from the general population has fallen – the mortality gap between those with and those without an SMI has increased.[14]

### What are the risk factors for people with SMI?
People with a severe mental illness are more likely than the general population to have risk factors for cardiovascular disease. They are also more likely

to have several risk factors, making their treatment more complex. Risk factors include that they are more likely to smoke and to be overweight. They are more likely to have diabetes, and more likely to have dyslipidaemia. Erectile dysfunction is a separate risk factor for cardiovascular disorder as is hyperprolactinaemia, both of which are complications of anti-psychotic medication. Erectile dysfunction – impotence – is also a complication of diabetes. Lithium treatment for bipolar affective disorder can also cause chronic kidney disease, a further risk factor for cardiovascular disorder.

### What are the effects of anti-psychotic medication?

Second generation anti-psychotic medication is recognised to induce factors that significantly increase the risk of cardiovascular disease. Studies show that it is the medication that plays a significant role in the development of these risk factors, rather than the illness for which the medication is prescribed. Anti-psychotic medication is also responsible for potentially fatal arrhythmias, including Torsades de Pointe. Finally, anti-psychotic medication causes venous thromboembolism, increasing the risk of both deep vein thrombosis and pulmonary embolism.

### What is the effect of lifestyle choices and social determinants of health?

People with severe mental illness access health care services less than others, and therefore are less likely to take up offers of cardiovascular prevention as frequently as others. Since people with severe mental illness are more likely to be unemployed, and homeless, they may be less able to afford medication that might be prescribed for the secondary prevention of cardiovascular disease. People with severe mental illness are more likely to smoke than the general population. Smoking increases the risk and severity of cardiovascular disease. There is some evidence that the prescribing of medication for tertiary prevention of cardiovascular disease following a myocardial infarction is less likely than the general population, for people with a severe mental illness.

### What is the effect of multi-morbidity?

People with severe mental illness are more likely to suffer from risk factors for cardiovascular disease, which includes diabetes. Diabetes is itself a risk factor for cardiovascular disease, and the complications of diabetes, such as renal failure and erectile dysfunction, are independent risk factors for cardiovascular disease. Smoking will exacerbate the effects of cardiovascular disease, the management of diabetes and the effects of thrombosis that is a side effect of anti-psychotic medication.

### What are the recommendations for clinical care?[15]

- In all countries, every person with SMI should have their cardiovascular risk assessed annually using an appropriate cardiovascular risk score algorithm. The FD should use whichever risk score algorithm is nationally or regionally recommended, e.g. SCORE, QRISK3.
- Where individuals with SMI have a high cardiovascular risk, they should be offered appropriate medication and interventions to reduce that risk, e.g. by adding aspirin, beta-blockers, angiotensin-converting enzyme inhibitors and/or statins, whilst acknowledging the risks associated with polypharmacy.
- Where individuals have sustained a cardiovascular event, they should be offered the same tertiary prevention treatment as people in the general population.
- In all countries, every person with SMI should be asked annually if they smoke tobacco, and where appropriate offered smoking cessation advice.
- In all countries people with SMI should be assessed for evidence of glucose dysregulation – by measuring the fasting blood glucose on an annual basis. For those who have developed diabetes, they should be offered the same treatment plans and follow-up as for those people with diabetes, but without severe mental illness.

## Alcohol and substance misuse in people with a severe mental illness

### What is the prevalence of the disorder in people with SMI?

A greater proportion of people with severe mental illness use harmful levels of alcohol than do people without a severe mental illness. Estimates suggest that between 35% and 80% of people with severe mental illness use harmful levels of alcohol. As a consequence, mortality rates for people with severe mental illness and alcohol misuse are significantly greater than for severe mental illness alone. (The alcohol hazard ratio for all-cause mortality in people with severe mental illness is 1.52.)[16,17]

People with schizophrenia have high rates of substance misuse, including tobacco, alcohol and cannabis.[18,19] They are also more likely to engage in substance misuse and high risk sexual behaviour which puts them at risk of Human Immunodeficiency Virus (HIV) infection, Hepatitis C or Hepatitis B. Up to 20% of people with a severe mental illness have been reported to have comorbid Hepatitis C; HIV has a reported prevalence of 7.8% (compared to 0.4% of people in the general population).

### What are the risk factors for people with SMI?

Harmful use of alcohol is a risk factor for readmission to a psychiatric hospital. However, long term follow-up of people with comorbid alcohol misuse and psychosis shows that they improve when they are provided with access to integrated treatment programmes.

There is an increased risk of any psychotic outcome in individuals who have ever used cannabis. The effect is dose related, with the greatest risk in those who use cannabis frequently. Starting smoking cannabis before the age of 15 increases the risk four-fold of developing psychosis.[20]

### What are the effects of anti-psychotic medication?

Treatment programmes for blood borne virus (BBV) disorders, although changing rapidly, are effective in people with severe mental illness. Some treatments can cause blood dyscrasias and should be used with caution in those people who are also taking anti-psychotic medication such as clozapine, that can also cause blood dyscrasias.

### What is the effect of lifestyle choices and social determinants of health – particularly seen in SMI?

The prevalence of Hepatitis C is higher (up to 40%) for those who are homeless and suffering from a severe mental illness, compared to those who are homeless without a severe mental illness.

### What is the effect of multi-morbidity?

Severe mental illness is a risk marker for acquiring BBV infections and comorbidity of psychosis and BBV infection worsens the prognosis for both conditions. A diagnosis of HIV is associated with an increased risk of developing psychosis, but a diagnosis of psychosis is not associated with an increased risk of HIV, unless there is comorbid substance misuse.

Amongst people with HIV, severe mental illness is six times more common than amongst those without HIV.

### Recommendations for clinical practice

- In all countries, people with SMI should be asked about their consumption of alcohol and offered appropriate advice to reduce harmful drinking. Advice should also include access to programmes that help to reduce harmful drinking, and access to programmes that support those who are homeless and in need of financial support.
- In all countries, people with SMI should be asked about behaviours that put them at risk of acquiring BBV diseases, and where appropriate be offered advice to reduce risk taking behaviour. Advice should include access to programmes that would support individuals to reduce risk taking behaviour, and access to programmes that support those who are homeless and in need of financial support.
- People should be offered blood tests to identify if liver function is normal, in particular, assessing liver damage secondary to alcohol, and BBV diseases. Abnormal results should also be reviewed to assess the possibility of non-alcoholic fatty liver disease, a significant risk in people with a metabolic syndrome and SMI.
- In those countries where some at risk groups are screened for BBV diseases), people with SMI should be offered the opportunity to be screened.
- Where available, people with SMI should be offered protection against Hepatitis B by vaccination.
- Where available, people with SMI who are HIV/AIDS positive or Hepatitis C positive should be offered treatment for these viral conditions, in the same way that people who are BBV positive but without SMI are offered treatment.

# Educational material

### Case study

Amir is a 38-year-old man in whom schizophrenia was diagnosed 22 years ago. There is no information in the clinical record as to his family history, or his social history, and no record of current employment status. There is no information about his smoking status. His records do reveal that he had numerous contacts with the practice nurse up until five months ago, and then nothing. The last few contacts were characterised by shouting, missing appointments, and generally chaotic behaviour.

During the consultation, Amir is quiet, polite and apologetic for his previous behaviour. He explains that he had become increasingly unwell mentally and had been admitted to hospital five months previously. His psychiatrist recently changed his medication to clozapine, and he feels much more settled and comfortable on this new treatment. He has been home for two weeks and has noticed that he is much more tired than previously and drinking water all the time. He mentioned this to his psychiatrist, who recommended that he see his family doctor.

*What should you focus on immediately?*
- Possible diagnosis of diabetes.
- Whether Amir smokes cigarettes.
- The discharge and communication process between secondary and primary care services.

All are important, but the immediate concern has to be around the possible development of diabetes.

You focus on the thirst and tiredness, cardinal features of diabetes. The family history is that mother and father had Type 2 diabetes. His father died of a heart attack aged 55 years. Amir's BMI has increased from 33 to 44 over the last two months. He has also started smoking again (he had the opportunity to buy take-away meals and cigarettes as part of his rehabilitation programme whilst on the ward).

*How do you diagnose diabetes?*
- Use HbA1c.
- Use fasting plasma glucose levels.

In general, either blood test is appropriate for diagnosing diabetes. However, WHO recommends that in a small number of situations the HbA1c may need to be supplemented by a fasting plasma glucose as well. This is because when patients start taking a drug like clozapine, the plasma glucose may rise very quickly – quicker than the HbA1c may rise, since it is dependent on the 90-day life cycle of the erythrocyte. In some circumstances therefore the HbA1c may be inappropriately low, and there is the danger of missing the diagnosis of diabetes especially if the clinical context is ignored.

At the next consultation you review the blood results, and a fasting blood glucose test confirms the diagnosis of diabetes. Country specific guidelines for newly diagnosed diabetics should be followed. These are likely to include:

- Information about diabetes;
- Advice about healthy eating, exercise and stopping smoking;
- Advice about influenza vaccination, pneumonia vaccination, Hepatitis B vaccination;
- Clinical examination to assess the baseline of target organs;
- Further blood tests to assess the lipid profile etc.

*What should you do next?*
- Start metformin.
- Reassess cardiovascular risk.
- Communicate the diagnosis to the psychiatrist.
- Advise Amir not to stop the clozapine.

All of these are important to consider. It is not clear when it is best to start metformin, and for most people with newly diagnosed diabetes, oral medication is not started at the time of diagnosis. However, in this case, Amir is already obese, and metformin is recommended for weight reduction as well as managing diabetes in people with SMI. Diabetes increases his cardiovascular risk significantly, and so ensuring that the diabetes is well controlled will be essential for his longer term care. Given the family history of both diabetes and early cardiovascular death, consideration will also need to be given to prescribing some cardioprotective medication including statins and antiplatelet medication.

Amir should be advised not to stop the clozapine as a way of managing the diabetes; this could clearly cause a relapse of his psychosis. His psychiatrist should also be informed of the diagnosis. This offers an opportunity for the psychiatrist to consider changing the clozapine for another medication that may be less diabetogenic, and for the mental health team to consider ways of improving communication between primary and secondary care.

## Multiple choice questions

1. Which of the following medications can be used to lose weight in people with a severe mental illness?

Alan Cohen and Kim Griswold

   a. Atorvastatin
   b. Aspirin
   c. Metformin
   d. Enalapril

2. Which one of the following side effects is *not* associated with second generation anti-psychotic medication?

   a. Hyperprolactinaemia
   b. Hyponatraemia
   c. Diabetogenic
   d. Obesogenic

3. Which one of the following is *not* a significant interaction between medications?

   a. Lithium and furosemide
   b. Clozapine and antiretrovirals
   c. Clozapine and antiplatelets
   d. Clozapine and ciprofloxacin

4. Which one of the following statements is true?

   a. Smoking cessation interventions are not effective in people with SMI.
   b. Smoking cessation interventions that use motivational interviewing techniques are effective in people with SMI.
   c. Smoking cessation interventions are expected to be as successful in people with SMI as for those in the general population without a mental illness.
   d. Smoking does not make diabetes worse in people with SMI.

5. Which one of the following is *not* a significant side effect of anti-psychotic medication?

   a. Potentially fatal arrhythmias
   b. Agranulocytosis
   c. Agranulocytopenia
   d. Thrombophilia

You will find the answers to these MCQs on page 171.

# References

1. World Health Organization: Fact Sheet. www.who.int/mental_health/management/info_sheet.pdf Accessed January 13, 2019.
2. United Nations: Transforming our world: the 2020 agenda for sustainable development. www.un.org.
3. Saxena S, Maj M. Physical health of people with severe mental disorders: leave no one behind. Editorial. *World Psychiatry* 2016, 16(1):1.
4. www.who.int/diabetes/global-report/en/ Accessed February 12, 2017.
5. www.who.int/mental_health/world-mental-health-day/paper_wfmh.pdf?ua=1 Accessed February 12, 2017.
6. Muench J, Hamer AM. Adverse effects of antipsychotic medications. *Ann Fam Practice* 2010, 81(5):617–622.
7. http://care.diabetesjournals.org/content/40/Supplement_1 Accessed February 13, 2017.
8. www.who.int/respiratory/en/ Accessed October 2015.
9. www.euro.who.int/en/health-topics/noncommunicable-diseases/chronic-respiratory-diseases/data-and-statistics Accessed October 2015.
10. www.who.int/respiratory/asthma/en/ Accessed October 2015.
11. www.who.int/topics/chronic_obstructive_pulmonary_disease/en/ Accessed October 2015.
12. www.euro.who.int/en/health-topics/disease-prevention/tobacco/data-and-statistics Accessed October 2015.
13. Smoking and Mental Health. A Joint Report of the Royal College of Physicians and the Royal College of Psychiatrists. London 2013.
14. www.euro.who.int/en/health-topics/noncommunicable-diseases/cardiovascular-diseases/data-and-statistics Accessed October 2016.
15. Piepoli MF, Hoes AW, Agewall S et al. European guidelines on cardiovascular disease prevention in clinical practice. *Eur Heart J* 2012, 33:1635–1701.
16. www.who.int/substance_abuse/en/.
17. Public health dimension of the world drug problem: a report by the Secretariat of the WHO Executive Board. 140th Session 28 Nov 2016, EB140/29.
18. www.who.int/substance_abuse/activities/gsrhua/en/.
19. Leposavic L, Dimitrijevic D, Dordevic S, et al. Comorbidity of harmful use of alcohol in population of schizophrenic patients. *Psychiatria Danubina* 2015, 27(1):84–89.
20. Drake R, Luciano A, Mueser K, et al. Longitudinal course of clients with co-occurring schizophrenia-spectrum and substance use disorders in urban mental health centers: a 7-year prospective study. *Schizophrenia Bul* 2016, 42(1):202–211.

*Information provided in this chapter is available as fact sheets, and the case study is available as a teaching tool. They can be downloaded from the WONCA website at: www.wonca.net/groups/WorkingParties/MentalHealth3/SMI.aspx*

Chapter 6

# MIGRANT MENTAL HEALTH CARE

Maria van den Muijsenbergh

# Key points

1.  Build a trustful relationship by providing person-centred, culturally competent care.
2.  Involve a professional interpreter or cultural navigator who is trusted by the patient. Adapt your language and any information provided to the patient's individual needs and situation.
3.  Get to know the migrant and their family/living circumstances.
4.  Be aware of cultural differences in health beliefs and expectations of health care, as well as shame or taboo relating to mental health problems.
5.  When a patient has a physical complaint, always perform a physical examination. If you suspect a mental health disorder, ask about the symptoms characteristic for this disorder.
6.  General lifestyle advice to support mental wellbeing is often relevant for migrants.
7.  Applying an integrative approach enables assessment of mental, physical and social issues, with a focus on strengthening resilience.
8.  Referral to a service with experience of caring for migrants with mental health problems is likely to ensure a culturally competent approach.
9.  Provide relevant psychoeducation, adapted to the language, culture and health literacy level of the patient.
10. Be aware of possible genetic differences in the metabolism of medication.

# Introduction

This chapter focuses on migrants: people who were born in another country than where they are living now. Much of the information in the chapter is also relevant to people from ethnic minorities.

Current estimates suggest that there are 244 million international migrants globally (or 3.3% of the world's population).[1] While the majority of individuals have migrated to countries within their region, a sizeable proportion migrate to high-income countries that are further afield. Economic factors are the major reason for migration, especially to high-income countries. Forced displacement is another important reason, leading to an estimated 25.4 million refugees in 2018.[2] As most high-income countries apply restrictive immigration policies, many immigrants are not granted legal permission to stay, but cannot or do not want to return to their country of origin. This results in an unknown number of irregular or undocumented migrants, who in most countries have limited or no access to social services and health care.

Though often healthy when they leave their country of origin, the health of many migrants deteriorates after arrival in the host country, with worse health and health outcomes over time, including mental health, than individuals of a similar social position in the guest country or in their country of origin.[3,4] Whilst differences in morbidity, violence and other unfavourable life experiences contribute to this high incidence, there is also growing evidence of the relationship between migration-related social problems, chronic stress and the rapid development of metabolic diseases, such as hypertension, being overweight, diabetes, anxiety and depression, particularly in refugees.[5] Migrants suffer disproportionately from the social determinants of poor mental health, including barriers to participating in society, perceived discrimination, social support and health literacy.[6] For instance, a higher prevalence of mental disorders in long-term refugees is associated with a lack of social integration and specifically with unemployment.[7]

As expressions of mental distress are highly influenced by cultural background, estimations of prevalence could be over- or underestimated by the standard diagnostic tools.[7] The prevalence of mental disorders in migrants shows a very high variation across different studies,[7,8] but all studies show higher rates for mood disorders, anxiety disorders and post traumatic stress disorder (PTSD). PTSD occurs specifically more often in refugee groups (9%–36% in refugees compared with 1%–2% in host populations).[7] The prevalence of depression in migrants varies between 5% and 44% compared to 8%–12% in the general population and for anxiety the prevalence in migrants varies from 4% to 40% compared to 5% in the general population. Also psychotic disorders are two to three times more prevalent in migrants than in host populations.[8]

Risk factors for developing mental disorders are rooted in social circumstances. Exposure to stressful events before departure or during travel and difficulties with settlement and integration/poor social integration in the host countries, particularly social isolation and unemployment, are associated with higher rates of mental disorders.[7] A recent large scale study showed higher prevalence of psychosis in migrants in 14 countries, even when adjusted for socioeconomic status. The authors suggest social exclusion and racism to explain this fact; for instance Ethiopian Jews are more at risk of developing psychosis than non-black Jewish immigrants in Israel.[9]

The risk of suicidal attempts and death by suicide is higher in some migrant groups, especially among non-European (south Asian and black African origin) immigrant women. Risk factors were found to be: language barriers, worrying about family back home and separation from family. The lack of information on health care systems, loss of status, loss of social network and acculturation were identified as possible triggers for suicidal behaviour.[10]

Misuse of alcohol and substance is also higher in migrants, especially refugees in difficult circumstances like refugee camps.[11]

## A trustful relationship and person-centred, culturally competent care

As in all patients, a person-centred approach optimises the mutual trust and understanding which benefits the outcomes of care.[12] Realisation of a person-centred approach in migrant populations requires knowledge of ethnic and cultural health differences and skills to communicate across linguistic and cultural differences.[13]

This approach is of particular importance in migrants where negative experiences with professionals and institutions may make building a therapeutic relationship of trust difficult. This means showing your empathy and interest, explaining your professional confidentiality (which might not have been experienced by people in their country of origin) and being aware of your own (implicit) bias regarding ethnicity, race, culture and religion. The 'medical gaze'[14] of doctors, caused by their training focused on biomedical pathology, can lead to medicalisation of behaviour and thoughts that differ from what they think to be normal. This might happen more easily when they encounter people from a different culture than their own.

## Importance of professional interpreters and cultural mediators

Professional interpreters improve patient–clinician interactions, provide a better patient experience and can also improve the outcome of psychological treatments.[7] Professional interpretation is of particular importance when talking about sensitive topics, e.g. mental health or violence experiences, where family and friends may not interpret accurately. Telephone or online interpretation services are increasingly available and can reduce costs. In some circumstances, e.g. small communities where people from the same language community know each other, telephone interpreters are to be preferred.

Cultural mediators can support migrants to effectively navigate through a health care system, if one assures that the mediator's gender and age fits with the patient's expectations. In many countries cultural mediators are available. These are migrants who know how the local health care systems work, speak the local language and support other migrants in their interactions with a health care system and professionals. Continuous presence of the same cultural mediator throughout a treatment process can help build trust and prevent patients from having to share their private stories with different mediators.[7]

# Get to know the migrant and their family/living circumstances

Primary care professionals should be aware of the social determinants and risk factors that influence the mental health of migrants: poverty, lack of social participation, perceived discrimination, limited health literacy due to language barriers and different expectations of health care. The only way to know this is to ask about it. This requires investing in at least two conversations (two 20 minute meetings should be sufficient). As trust building between the family physician and patient is of the utmost importance, at least one of these 'getting to know you' conversations should be held by the doctor personally. The follow-up intake conversation could also be performed by a practice nurse or social worker in the practice. In the Netherlands, the Dutch college of General Practitioners (NHG) has developed a format for items to be assessed in every new patient, in order to have sufficient information on the patients' context to provide person-centred care[15] (see Table 6.1).

Sensitive topics including experiences of violence should only be asked about if sufficient trust has been built up. In the first consultation with your patient, it is best to explore the reason for the encounter and to provide the patient space to talk about this. Then, before deepening your history taking, explain that you first want to get to know the patient better, in order to more effectively answer their question and help them.

It is important to assess the level of literacy of your patient in order to adjust your information. Patients with limited (health-)literacy skills are best helped if you:

- Speak slowly and take time for the conversation;
- Use simple words and avoid medicalised vocabulary;

**Table 6.1** Assessment of the new migrant patient

---

**First conversation – getting-to-know-you conversation**
**If possible, arrange for a professional interpreter**
**Provide the following information**
**Emphasise professional confidentiality**
**How your health clinic works (making an appointment, length of consultation slot, out-of-hours service etc.)**
The concept of family medicine (specialist training, for all problems, evidence-based care)
The role of all members of the clinical team, e.g. when practice assistants perform triage when a patient wants to make an appointment
That you want to ask a range of personal questions, in order to get to know the person and their life. Emphasise that the patient only needs to answer questions they feel comfortable in doing so.
**Language**
What is your mother tongue?
What languages can you understand or speak?
What language do you speak at home?
What languages are you able to read? And write?
**Do you want an interpreter?**
How often do you need help to fill out forms? (asking about low literacy)
**Country of origin**
**Where were you born and raised?**
Where are your parents from?
In the case of migration:

- How long have you been in this country?
- With whom did you come to this country (family, alone, friends)?
- What was your reason for migrating?

**Living circumstances and family**
**Is there anyone who can act as a contact person for you? If so, which language does she/he speaks?**
Where do you live? Is this temporary?
With whom do you share your home?
In the case of homelessness:

- Where do you usually sleep?

Do you have children?

- If so, what are their names, how old are they and where do they live?

Do you stay in contact with family members?

- If so, where do they live?

**Education and work**
**How many years did you go to school? Where? Did you get any certificates?**
Have you been taught a specific profession?
Are you employed now? If so, what kind of job do you have? Is it temporary or permanent?
What jobs have you been doing, in your country of origin or here?

---

**Table 6.1** (Cont.)

Are you on social welfare?

Do you have any financial worries? Do you have any financial debts?

**Religion**

**Is there any religion of importance to you?**

**First intake – medical information**

**Medical information: general**

**Allergies**

**Substance use: smoking, alcohol, recreational drugs**

Diseases that run in the family (often not know by migrants)?

**Medical information: problem list**

**Have you ever stayed in a hospital? If so, when and why?**

Have you ever been seriously ill? If so, when and what, are you fully recovered?

Are there any diseases you suffer from? Now, or chronically, or for which you take medication?

Do you take medication? If so, what and when?

Do you take any herbs or traditional medication?

**Medical information: infectious diseases**

**Tuberculosis screening**

**Hepatitis B/C?**

**HIV?**

**Vaccinations**

**Second conversation to obtain more personal information**

**Culture**

**What do you value most/think is most important in your culture?**

With whom do you usually talk about worries or illness?

Who do you ask for advice or help?

**Life events**

**How did you come to this country?**

Have you ever lost family or friends? Do you want to talk about that?

Have you ever experienced violence? Physically? Or mentally (people criticising you or threatening you). Have you ever had a bad sexual experience or been forced to have sex?

Have you even been harassed by the police? Have you ever spent time in jail?

**Integration**

**Do you feel at home in this country?**

Do you have any friends or acquaintances from this (the new) country?

Do you feel excluded from society? From your community? Have you ever experienced discrimination?

Source: adapted from van den Muijsenbergh & Oosterberg 2016[15]

- Support your information audio-visually (pictures, YouTube movies etc.);
- Limit the amount of information to the essentials;
- At the end of the consultation, ask the patient to tell you what you have discussed (teach-back).

## Cultural differences in beliefs about mental health and differences in health care expectations

Different cultures and communities exhibit or explain symptoms in various ways. For example, uncontrollable crying and headaches are symptoms of panic attacks in some cultures, while difficulty breathing may be the primary symptom in other cultures. Knowledge about such distinctions can help health care workers to ask the patient about the meaning of their symptoms, and thus more accurately diagnose and effectively treat them. Specific beliefs about mental phenomena and psychological distress often seen in migrants relate to supernatural explanations. Some cultures, e.g. Moroccan, may be relatively accepting of 'hearing voices', while others may perceive it as a psychiatric symptom, e.g. Dutch. Several culture-bound expressions of anxiety and culture-bound syndromes are detailed within the appendices of the DSM-5 classification.[16] Be also aware of your own (implicit) cultural bias and 'medical gaze' (see above).

Cultural expectations influence how mental health care is regarded. Rituals, traditional herbal medicines, priests or traditional healers play an important role in many cultures, however these are often not mentioned spontaneously by migrants. It is important to ask about them. Tensions may occur if patients believe they are seriously mentally or physically ill and expect a more or less specific pharmacological or psychological treatment, which the clinician does not suggest or provide.[7]

## Diagnosing mental health problems and screenings instruments

Often migrants describe major depression or other mental health problems in terms of physical symptoms (pain, fatigue or other nonspecific symptoms). Even if you suspect a mental health problem, always perform a physical examination. Doing so will reassure a patient that the origin of their complaints is not a physical illness. If mental health symptoms including depressed mood, fears, self-harm and suicidal ideation are not mentioned, you may have to specifically ask about them. As shame or taboo can play a role, it often helps to start with general questions about life and wellbeing before moving on to more specific questions related to mental health. Even then, many migrants are not used to discussing their feelings in the same words as doctors do (in some languages, e.g. Turkish, there may not be a native word for 'depressed'; instead the word 'karamsar' is used, meaning black or dark).

When talking about suicide, it is recommended[17] to approach the topic gradually, by first asking about other aspects of distress and posing questions that may make it easier for a person to answer honestly, for example:

- 'Some people with similar problems have told me that they felt life was not worth living.'
- 'Do you sometimes go to sleep wishing that you might not wake up in the morning?'

If mental health disorders are suspected, existing screening instruments like the PHQ-9 can be used to screen for depression (www.uspreventiveservices taskforce.org/Home/ … /218).

For global screening of mental health problems, including PTSD, the RHS-15 could be used. This instrument was specifically designed for and validated on newly arrived refugees with items derived from existing and valid instruments used on similar populations. It is available in several languages; it can be administered in a relatively short time and is easily understandable for people of different educational levels. Furthermore, it measures several relevant mental health constructs related to emotional distress typical for refugee and migrant populations.[18] The RHS-15 is an open access tool and may be obtained at www. uppdragpsykiskhalsa.se/verktyg/rhs-refugee-health-screener/.

Routine screening for exposure to traumatic events should be undertaken with caution. Pushing for disclosure of traumatic events in well-functioning individuals may result in more harm than good.[19]

Be aware of the higher risk of alcohol and substance use among migrants in difficult living circumstances like refugee camps, and ask about this.[11] Think of the use of Kat in migrants from the horn of Africa.

## The importance of integrated care

Given the importance of social determinants in the development of both physical and mental health problems, an integrated approach is important. By this we mean that the physical, emotional, mental, social concerns of migrant patients are assessed and if possible addressed.[7] For instance, many migrants, even those living in high-income countries, have financial problems (in the Netherlands 75% of Syrian refugees and 83% of Eritrean refugee families are living below the poverty line).

Knowing where to find and how to refer to social care, welfare and specialised services for particularly vulnerable subgroups (e.g. those exposed to torture, victims of human trafficking) can help to realise this integrative approach. Also, acquaintance with volunteer or migrant representative organisations can help to find adequate support for migrants, especially those who have difficulty navigating the health care system.

# Referral and treatment of mental health disorders

Most migrants with mental disorders do not require different interventions from those that are commonly provided for people with mental disorders in the general host population. Evidence-informed guidelines apply to refugees and migrants as to any other group.[7] Most migrants exposed to stressful events are likely to have developed resilience. Many have existing strengths and skills or develop new abilities in the host country that can help them to achieve social integration and be a resource for the country that they live in.

Usual treatments like EMDR (Eye Movement Desensitisation and Reprocessing) have often not been studied in migrant groups, but good experiences in migrants exist with 'narrative exposure therapy', which helps patients to develop a chronological narrative of their life story with a focus on the traumatic experiences, in order to transform fragmented reports of the traumatic experiences into a coherent narrative.[7]

As many barriers exist for migrants to effectively access mental health care, a thoughtful referral and an integrative approach are necessary (see Table 6.2).

# Psychoeducation

Providing relevant psychoeducation is important as many migrants are not familiar with the effects of stress, trauma and grief on the mind and body. It can help migrants to understand the sometimes overwhelming feelings that naturally arise from the many stressors they face. For example, people may

**Table 6.2** Principles of successful referral for migrant mental health care

### Active care coordination

1. Direct referral to a Mental Health (MH) provider (e.g. making appropriate referral on a client's behalf, assisting with scheduling of the first appointment).
2. Good communication between referring and receiving providers (e.g. discussing referral, case-specific education, sharing case files and assessment results, consultation and ongoing contact after initial referral).
3. Good case management (e.g. help in identifying appropriate services, providing information on MH services and how to access them, coordinating discharge planning after psychiatric hospitalisation).

### Establishing trust and identifying mental health symptoms

4. Trust developed through family or ethnic community leaders, health or non-health providers (e.g. referral made by non-MH providers, such as primary care providers, nurses, language learning programmes, interpreters).
5. Proactive identification of MH symptoms (e.g. accessing MH services through staff not directly involved with MH delivery).
6. Access to embedded MH or referral coordinators (e.g. MH providers embedded in health or non-health settings).

### Proactive resolutions of access barriers

7. Psychoeducation (e.g. about the process and benefits of accessing MH services, differences between Western and cultural specific MH concepts, roles of different health providers, payment for MH services).
8. Interpreters (e.g. interpreter support available for MH appointments and referral).
9. Transportation (e.g. providers help arrange transportation for MH appointments such as medical taxi drivers).
10. Follow-up (e.g. reminders about the appointment, contacting the client after the initial appointment to ask how it went, offering additional help such as rescheduling when necessary).

### Culturally responsive care

11. Knowledge of refugees' culture (e.g. adapting treatment to be culturally relevant, using appropriate language to discuss MH and wellbeing).
12. Flexibility to meet in client's home (e.g. because of fear of being stigmatised).
13. Multidisciplinary care (e.g. advocacy and assistance to receive additional services and resources, helping with paperwork for medical assistance).

Source: adapted from Ajdukovic et al, 2017[17]

experience changes in sleep and eating habits, quickly break into tears or can be easily irritated. It can be helpful to reassure people of the normality of many of these reactions and provide simple ways to cope with distress and negative feelings. Providing brief and practical information in an appropriate language that people in this situation can understand is helpful. Information should use everyday language and avoid using clinical terms like traumatised or PTSD.

## Genetic differences in the metabolism of medication

Although genetic variation between individuals within an ethnic group can be broad, some characteristics are more common in specific groups. This is of relevance in the metabolism of some medications involving the CYP450 pathway, including antidepressants and antipsychotics.[20] 'Slow metabolism', resulting in (side-)effects of drugs at a lower than usual dosage, occur in 10%–25% of people originating from Asia. It is possible to test the blood for CYP450 polymorphism, but for daily practice you can manage by applying the following rule in migrants from Turkey or eastwards: 'start low (half of the usual dose of antidepressant), rise slow'. 'Ultra fast metabolism' on the other hand resulting in a lack of effect in otherwise effective dosage, occurs in 30% of people of Ethiopian descent and in 20% of people originating from the Arabian Middle East. If, for instance, an antipsychotic drug does not have the expected effect in this group, you could increase the dose before changing to another drug.

People with West or Middle African roots (like many Afro-Americans and people from the West Indies) are more likely to develop dyskinesia when taking antipsychotics.[21]

## Implications for service delivery

Accessing care is often difficult for migrants due to problems shared by all migrant groups. These include structural barriers relating to the system (limitation of entitlements for certain groups, waiting lists and unclear procedures), barriers in the accessibility of available services (language barriers, transportation costs and out of pocket payments, lack of information about the health care system and fear of unknown (financial) consequences), barriers arising from the patient–provider contact such as language barriers and cultural differences in explanatory models of mental distress and in health care expectations.[7] A recent review revealed a further important barrier in that many migrants do not identify their symptoms as medical.[22] They often believe the illness to be part of their destiny and therefore rely on alternative forms of support such as healing through praying or herbs, or seeking social support among members of their community.[16]

Stigma through previous experiences of not having been taken seriously by health care providers, perceived or actual discrimination and privacy concerns act as social barriers to care seeking. Professionals often experience complex referral procedures and eligibility criteria for migrants to access mental health care. Sometimes migrants expect more medication than offered, while some individuals, their family, or faith leaders have concerns about medication and will not take it.

Efforts to overcome these barriers must take place at various levels:

1.  Policy level:

    *   The right to health care for all should be guaranteed by ensuring equal entitlements for all migrants and eliminating structural financial barriers.

2.  Health care organisations:

    *   Simplify administrative and care procedures;
    *   Provide clear, easy to understand multi-lingual information on any procedures or treatment;
    *   Provide interpreter services.

3.  Individual health care providers:

    *   Work on creating a trustful relationship with their patients. This has been identified as essential to the (continued) use of services. This requires a person-centred culturally sensitive approach as described above. Personal continuity of care is an important element in this.
    *   Advocate for equitable and accessible mental health care services.

4.  Migrant communities and organisations:

    *   Identify key persons and cultural mediators;
    *   Provide information on the local health care system and on common mental health issues;
    *   Provide social support alongside support to visit mental health care professionals;
    *   Work on stigma within their community;
    *   Advocate for adequate support and services.

Maria van den Muijsenbergh

# Educational material

### Case study

On a busy Monday morning Naima enters your consultation room. You know her quite well. She is a young North African woman, very active in her community. Consultations with her are always easy. But today, she is not alone. With her comes a girl you have never seen before. She looks to the floor and gives a very weak handshake; she does not say a word. She looks very sad. Naima tells you her name is Latifa, she is 20 years old and she is not feeling at all well. Naima did not know who to turn to as Latifa has just arrived in your city. Originaly she is from Egypt, Naima thinks; they met at the Mosque, where Latifa was brought by her aunt who was very worried about her. Naima had tried to speak with Latifa, but got the impression that she was very afraid and ill. She does not know if Latifa has health insurance, but she does know that the girl needs help, right now.

*If Latifa does not have health insurance, are you obliged to help her? Yes or no.*
Yes. According to medical ethics, as a doctor you must help all patients regardless of their background or financial status.

*It is Monday morning, your waiting room is filled with patients. You clearly have very limited time now to handle this. Your practice list is already overcapacity and you had agreed with your colleagues not to accept new patients. What would be the best strategy?*
  a. Be honest and tell Naima, you are very sorry but you cannot help her. She should find another doctor for Latifa.
  b. Start the consultation to get it over with as soon as possible.
  c. Explain why you cannot help her now and ask her to come back at another time.
  d. Make a new specific appointment as soon as possible.

As migrants often feel rejected, and Latifa clearly needs help, it is important you let her feel you want to help. A therapeutic relationship requires trust to be built. In order to make sure she and Naima understand this, and that you have a mutual understanding of the procedure, you should be very specific about the new appointment, and make sure it fits their schedule as well as yours.

You understand this is an urgent problem, but you will need time to explore what is going on. Therefore, you ask Naima if she and Latifa can come back at lunchtime, to have more time for the consultation. They agree and come back a few hours later.

*Latifa will probably not speak your language, as she has just arrived from Egypt. Naima probably does. What would be the best strategy to handle this?*
    a.  Ask Naima to translate.
    b.  Call a professional interpreter and ask Naima to leave the room.
    c.  Call a professional interpreter and ask Naima to stay.
    d.  Use Google Translate to ensure maximum anonymity of the interpreter.

The best option is to request a professional interpreter and ask through this interpreter whether Latifa wishes for Naima to stay. Often this is the case as the patient will feel supported and advocated for by the presence of a compatriot who also understands the language and culture of the host country.

With a male Arabic interpreter on the phone you start your conversation with Latifa.

*Could the interpreter be a problem? Yes or no.*
If Latifa has problems that are related to sexual or reproductive health, she may find this hard to share with a male interpreter. If you do not know a patient, then try to find a gender congruent interpreter.

Latifa explains that she does not feel well, her belly aches, she cannot eat, she has lost her appetite and she is very tired. This started when she arrived in your country. She thinks she might have caught a local disease.

All your further questions do not reveal any indication for a gastrointestinal or gynaecological disease.

You are increasingly convinced that Latifa is suffering from a mental health problem. Therefore, you explain you don't believe she has an infection and you don't perform a physical examination.

*Is this right? Yes or no.*
To convince Latifa that she does not have such an illness, and to give her the feeling you have taken her seriously, you should examine her abdomen and undertake appropriate investigations, e.g. blood pressure. Only after specific reassurance that her body is healthy will you be able to explain that sometimes the body feels ill because of stress or other problems, and continue with your mental health questions.

To your surprise, when asking Latifa if she feels depressed, she says no, although she looks very depressed.

*How can you explain this?*

    a.   She is not depressed and your impression has been influenced by your implicit bias, thinking women who will not look you in the face and smile will have to be depressed.

    b.   She does not know the word depressed, not even in her own language.

    c.   She feels ashamed about wrong feelings.

    d.   She does not want Naima to know this, for fear of the stigma of mental health problems in the community.

These could all be true; you should ask more questions, probably without Naima in the room, to get a deeper understanding of her problems.

In keeping with your regular practice, you are thinking about using the PHQ-9 to assess for depression.

*Can you use this questionnaire? Yes or no*

Yes, the PHQ-9 is valid for migrants, if you administer it in their own language, and make sure the patient understands all questions by asking them to tell you what they mean.

You remember that it is always important to get to know the context of the patient and ask her about her life circumstances and her life in Egypt.

Naima tells you she had a 'bad' experience in Egypt with a man, and her family had sent her away to stay with her aunt in your country. Since this experience she does not sleep, even though she is very tired, she is easily startled by noise and loses her temper very quickly. Now Naima adds that she overheard her aunt say to the Imam that it is the work of a Djin.

*How should you react to this information?*

    a.   In order to help Latifa to find adequate care, it is important you make very clear Djins do not exist.

    b.   You ask Latifa what she thinks about Djins.

    c.   You ignore the information and go on asking about the 'bad' experience in Egypt.

    d.   You say that you know about Djins and how Imams can help sometimes to get rid of them.

It would be best to ask Latifa about the Djin. Ignoring or rejecting the existence of Djins will probably harm the confidence Latifa will have in you, preventing you from gaining further information on what they are going to do about the Djin, and will probably form a barrier against effective help. Stating that you know about Djins may seem like a means of building trust, however doing so assumes you know what Latifa has experienced. It is always best to ask the patient what they think about culturally influenced health beliefs.

After a lengthy conversation, Latifa begins to speak more and makes some eye contact. You are convinced she suffers from PTSD and you suspect sexual violence. You do not wish to ask about this in a first consultation. You want to refer her to a mental health specialist with expertise on migrant women and sexual violence. In keeping with your standard practice, you make an electronic referral to a large mental health care service you work with, and tell Latifa that she will receive an invitation for an assessment within that service within four weeks.

*Is this a good way to refer? Yes or no*
This isn't a good way to refer. The chances are high that Latifa will never arrive, or the therapy will not start properly. The appointment letter may not reach her as she may change address or may not have anyone in the house able to read the letter. She will not know where to go, or may not have enough money for public transport. She may not trust the 'unknown person' who will conduct the assessment. The mental health care service may not have an interpreter available, and she will not be able to understand the paperwork required for further care.

Ideally, for a vulnerable migrant like Latifa you arrange a 'warm' referral. You call the psychologist you want her to be allocated to and make a personal appointment, if possible while Latifa is still in your room, so she hears you speaking with the therapist. Although in many systems procedures will make this impossible, it is worthwhile to discuss this with the MH service you are collaborating with.

An alternative is to involve a 'peer supporter', a migrant speaking her mother tongue who can act as a navigator through the system, and accompany her to appointments. Check if the appointment fits in with her agenda, if an interpreter will be available, and if Latifa understands where and when she has to go, and if she is able to do so.

Make a follow-up appointment to get to know her better, and to check how she is doing while waiting for the therapist. During that appointment, you could ask about her medical history, and include in this the question about if she has had a bad sexual experience. To introduce this delicate issue, it is important to 'normalise' it, for instance by saying: 'As I know that many women have suffered from bad sexual experiences, and that these experiences can damage your health, I always ask new patients if they have ever suffered from a bad sexual experience, for instance being touched by a man you did not want, or have sex without protection.'

If sexual violence has taken place, do not forget to ask about symptoms of sexually transmitted infections and possible pregnancy. Explain to Latifa what PTSD is, and why she is experiencing the nasty things she feels.

# Further reading and e-resources

## Further reading

- Bhugra D, Gupta S, Bhui K, et al. WPA guidance on mental health and mental health care in migrants. *World Psychiatry* 2011, 10:2–10.
- Giacco D, Priebe S. Mental health care for adult refugees in high-income countries. *Epidemiol Psychiatr Sci* 2018, 27:109–16.
- Close C, Kouvonen A, Bosqui T, et al. The mental health and wellbeing of first generation migrants: a systematic-narrative review of reviews. *Glob Health* 2016, 12:47.
- Nosè M, Ballette F, Bighelli I, et al. Psychosocial interventions for post-traumatic stress disorder in refugees and asylum seekers resettled in high-income countries: systematic review and meta-analysis. *PLOS One* 2017, 12: e0171030.
- WHO Regional Office for Europe. Mental health promotion and mental health care in refugees and migrants. Copenhagen, 2018 (Technical guidance on refugee and migrant health).

## e-resources

- www.pharos.nl/infosheets/voorlichtingsmateriaal-over-psychische-gezondheid-voor-asielzoekers-en-vluchtelingen/
- http://eur-human.uoc.gr/module-5-part-1-2mental-health-issues-of-refugees/ Rapid assessment mental health triage tool, developed within the EUR-HUMAN project
- Psychological First Aid for Children (Save the Children) https://resourcecentre. savethechildren.se/library/save-children-psychological-first-aid-training-manual-child-practitioners
- Psychoeducation leaflet for children. *http://mhpss.net/?get=83%2F1305723318-2._Brochure_on_support_to.pdf*
- Self-help book for Syrian men facing crisis and displacement: https://publications. iom.int/books/self-help-booklet-men-facing-crisis-and-displacement-0
- Psychoeducation leaflet on coping. *http://mhpss.net/?get=83/1305723483-1. _Brochure_on_stress_and_coping.pdf*
- www.moodcafe.co.uk/mental-health-info/trauma-and-abuse/post-traumatic-stress-disorder.aspx

# References

1. International Organization for Migration (IOM). World migration report 2018. IOM, Geneve 2017. www.iom.int/wmr/world-migration-report-2018

2. UNHCR. Figures at a glance. www.unhcr.org/ph/figures-at-a-glance (accessed 25 February 2019).

3. Rechel B, Mladovsky P, Ingleby D, et al. Migration and health in an increasingly diverse Europe. *Lancet* 2013, 381:1235–1245.

4. Hadgkiss EJ, Renzaho AM. The physical health status, service utilisation and barriers to accessing care for asylum seekers residing in the community: a systematic review of the literature. *Aust Health Rev* 2014, 38:142–159.

5. Schulz AJ, House JS, Israel BA, et al. Relational pathways between socioeconomic position and cardiovascular risk in a multi-ethnic urban sample: complexities and their implications for improving health in economically disadvantaged populations. *J Epidemiol Community Health* 2008, 62:638–646.

6. Hirani K, Payne D, Mutch R, et al. Health of adolescent refugees resettling in high-income countries. *Arch Dis Child* 2015. doi: 10.1136/archdischild-2014-307221.

7. WHO Regional Office for Europe. *Mental health promotion and mental health care in refugees and migrants.* Copenhagen: WHO Europe 2018.

8. Close C, Kouvonen A, Bosqui T, et al. The mental health and wellbeing of first generation migrants: a systematic-narrative review of reviews. *Globalization and Health* 2016, 12:47.

9. Selten J-P, van der Von E, Termorshuizen F. Migration and psychosis: a meta-analysis of incidence studies. *Psychol Med* 2019. doi: https://doi.org/10.1017/S0033291719000035.

10. Forte A, Trobia F, Gualtieri F, et al. Suicide risk among immigrants and ethnic minorities: a literature overview. *Int J Environ Res Public Health* 2018, 15:1438.

11. Horyniak D, Melo JS, Farrell RM, Ojeda VD. Strathdee SA epidemiology of substance use among forced migrants: a global systematic review. *PLOS ONE* 2016, 11(7): e0159134.

12. Eklund JH, Holmström IK, Kumlin T, et al. 'Same same or different?' A review of reviews of person-centered and patient-centered care. *Patient Educ Couns* 2019, 102(1): 3–11.

13. Seeleman C, Suurmond J, Stronks K. Cultural competence: a conceptual framework for teaching and learning. *Med Educ* 2009, 43:229–237.

14. Foucault M. *The birth of the clinic: an archaeology of medical perception.* University Press of France, Paris, 1963.

15. Van Den Muijsenbergh METC, Oosterberg E (eds). Zorg voor laaggeletterden, migranten en social kwetsbaren in de huisartsenpraktijk (Care for low literate, migrant or socially vulnerable people in General Practice). NHG (Dutch College for General Practitioners)/ Pharos, Utrecht, The Netherlands 2016. pp.103–104.

16. American Psychiatry Association. *Diagnostic and statistical manual of mental disorders.* 5th ed. 2013, Psychiatry Association Publishing, Washington, D.C. and USA. pp. 833–837.

17. Ajdukovic D, Bakic H, Lionis C et al on behalf of the EUR-HUMAN research consortium. Protocol for assessment of mental health problems. Deliverable 1 Eur-Human project. http://eur-human.uoc.gr/wp-content/uploads/2017/05/D5_1_Protocol_with_procedures_ tools_for_rapid_assessment_provision.pdf

18. Kaltenbach E, Härdtner E, Hermenau K, et al. Efficient identification of mental health problems in refugees in Germany: the Refugee Health Screener. *Eur J Psychotraumatol* 2017, 8(sup2):1389205. doi: 10.1080/20008198.2017.1389205.

19. Canadian collaboration for immigrant and refugee health: guidelines and e-courses. www.ccirhken.ca/

20. Ingelman-Sundberg M. Pharmacogenetics of cytochrome P450 and its applications in drug therapy: the past, present and future. *Trends Pharmacol Sci* 2004, 25(4):193–200.

21. van Harten PN, Hoek HW, Matroos GE, van Os J. Incidence of tardive dyskinesia and tardive dystonia in African Caribbean patients on long-term antipsychotic treatment: the Curaçao extrapyramidal syndromes study V. *J Clin Psychiatry* 2006, 67(12):1920–1927.

22. Van der Boor C, White R. Barriers to accessing and negotiating mental health services in asylum seekers and refugee populations: the application of the candidacy framework, review article. *Journal of Immigrant and Minority Health.* doi:10.1007/s10903-019-00929-y. Published online 23 August 2019.

Chapter 7

# MENTAL HEALTH OF YOUNG PEOPLE

Jane Roberts and Christopher Dowrick

This chapter offers guidance to front line family doctors and primary care nurses on how to offer a friendly and effective interaction for young people with mental health problems.

# Key points

1. Prepare your working environment.
2. Put the young person at ease.
3. Clarify confidentiality.
4. Open the conversation in the context of the young person's life.
5. Scope out any possible risk areas.
6. Undertake an appropriate physical examination.
7. Offer basic psychoeducation.
8. Offer simple relaxation techniques and strategies for de-stressing.
9. Signpost for support.
10. Agree a follow-up plan.

# Introduction

Historically, adolescence was defined by WHO as the period between 10 and 19 years of age. In more recent years WHO have adopted a less formally defined term – 'young people' – to refer to people aged between 10 and 24 years. We will use this term throughout this chapter.

Adolescence is a unique life transition whereby young people must distance themselves from adult influences if their neuro-cognitive maturation is to be complete. At the same time they must navigate new psychosexual, social, economic and political challenges unknown to their parents' generation. Decisions made in these formative years may have life-long implications.

There has been an unprecedented increase in the total number of young people. The current generation comprises 1.8 billion globally. This represents more than 25% of the world's population and is the largest generation of young people ever recorded. More than 90% of young people live in low to middle income countries where, because of higher fertility rates, they constitute a higher proportion of the population.[1]

Where young people's health has been jeopardised by inadequate education, by violence at home or in their community, by poverty, conflict or forced migration, their assets are compromised and their life chances diminished. This in turn means their contribution to a happy and healthy society is reduced.

Mental health problems are the biggest health problem faced by young people yet one of the most under-resourced and least developed. Most mental health problems begin during adolescence and continue into adulthood. There is evidence of a global rise in the order of 10%–20% of children and adolescents experiencing mental health problems.[2] Young people growing up in poverty are recognised as being at high risk, due to additional burdens of stress which compromise healthy psychosocial development.

Young people are at high risk of suicide with one third of countries showing the highest rates in people aged under 25 years. In China and India suicide is the leading cause of death.[3] UK based studies reveal 3 in 4 young people with 'problem behaviours', anxiety or depression receive no help; the greatest gap between mental health prevalence and service use occurs amongst people under 25; access to treatment and support is worsening with providers reporting increasing complexity and severity of problems amongst young people seeking help; 77% of young people are in debt by age 21.[4] There are also high rates of increase in self harm.[5]

Investing in young people's health and wellbeing strengthens a country's assets. However, in general, this has not been a priority in health care planning or education. Increasing attention has focused on the first 1000 days of life, and the lack of interest in adolescence has resulted in the least progress being seen in young people's health than for any other life stage. The increased disease burden for young people arises from preventable and treatable problems including HIV and other infectious diseases, poor sexual and reproductive health, undernutrition and unintentional injury. The negative consequences of this are far reaching, with young people being both the parents of the next generation and the carers of the oldest generation.

Young people face multiple challenges and burdens which are new to this generation as it navigates change occurring at a rapid rate. Pressures include dealing with intergenerational and cultural conflict which leads to relationship stressors and family difficulties; against a background of increasing uncertainty. Academic pressures to excel have risen yet are coupled with decreasing and unreliable employment opportunities.

Investing in young people's physical and mental health, because the two are always inseparable, is a win-win strategy where everyone benefits. Investing in adolescence yields the triple dividend of 'benefits during adolescence, across the life course, and into the next generation.'[6]

The maelstrom of adolescent development, which rejects adult involvement and yet at the same time needs a compassionate steer, leaves its mark in the family doctor's consulting room. Young people presenting with emotional distress, challenging, disturbing or risky behaviour can leave a health care practitioner feeling uncertain about how best to proceed, anxious about their competence and knowledge base and lacking in confidence.[7] Adolescent emotional distress presents professional challenges to family doctors who feel ill equipped and inadequately prepared to address young peoples' problems as they present in the consulting room.

We know that the social determinants of adolescent health lie outside the remit of medicine and the causes of poor mental health in young people under the age of 25 cannot be solved with a medical approach alone. However, family doctors remain a relatively accessible source of help for young people. Responses can be therapeutic and beneficial in addressing emotional distress, if practitioners are supported in their professional development.

# Explaining the key points

### 1. Prepare your working environment.

Confidentiality and a respectful attitude are fundamental dimensions of truly youth-friendly health services, in addition to more practical factors relating to accessibility and availability such as location and cost.

How easily can young people access their family doctor? What is the level of staff training and confidence around confidentiality? How well do they understand how young people's needs are different from those of older patients? Does the consulting environment take into account the needs of young people? Are there posters describing confidentiality? Are there offers of local services?

For young people to feel at ease in the health setting there need to be visible signs that they have been considered as a distinct social group with needs which are different from adults. Evidence that consultations will take place in a safe, comfortable and welcoming space begins with the reception area and staff who greet young people kindly and professionally. This might be achieved by a display of posters of youth services, a décor which is fresh and attractive, and furniture which is modern.

Recommendations for both the value of and the nature of youth-friendly services have largely developed from action based research which has its origins in co-constructed studies where young people have been equal partners in the research activity from the outset. Tylee et al. published a seminal paper which presents key models of youth-friendly health provision and reviews the supporting evidence for the efficacy of such models on young people's health.[8]

Regarding the work environment, they recommend:

- Ensuring privacy (including a discrete entrance);
- Ensuring consultations occur after a short waiting time, with or without an appointment, and (where necessary) swift referral;
- Lack of stigma;
- An appealing and clean environment;
- An environment that ensures physical safety;
- Providing information in a variety of methods.

They note that 'many of these initiatives have not been appropriately assessed. Appropriate controlled assessments of the effect of youth-friendly health-service models on young people's health outcomes should be the focus of future research agendas.'[8] They will also need financial investment in youth mental health, which is not widely seen globally.

### 2. Put the young person at ease.

Putting the young person at ease is the primary task of any family doctor, although not easy in a time-pressured, task-oriented environment, They will need time and likely several meetings to gain confidence.

It can feel impossible when a young person is accompanied by an anxious, or frustrated parent, or when the young person has not chosen to be present but has been co-coerced into attending. However, unless steps are taken to diffuse any tension and to demonstrate a desire to genuinely listen to the young person, the consultation will have minimum impact and may be counter-productive.

Positive and welcoming non-verbal behaviour is pivotal, remembering to keep a relaxed face and a genuine smile being key. Often when we are unsure how to proceed as doctors we can gravitate to medical terminology: this is to be avoided with young people; not out of a desire to over simplify but to use language which is familiar and reassuring and allow for the explanation of more challenging concepts.

### 3. Clarify confidentiality.

Confidentiality is a vital issue for young people. They will be asking themselves who they can trust with their most intimate fears and experiences.

As family doctors, we need to be very clear about our lines of inquiry, and about who else might need to be involved if there is concern about their safety. It is important to be explicit about the Three Harms Confidentiality caveat that confidentiality will only be broken if the doctor is concerned that the patient is at risk of harming themselves, harming someone else or being harmed by someone else.

Having explicit posters summarising the tenets of confidentiality displayed in the waiting area are useful resources to remind staff and young people alike of best practice. Staff confidence on this topic is best achieved by in-house staff professional educational development, and is addressed in the section on 'Service delivery'.

### 4. Open the conversation in the context of the young person's life.

Youth mental health is influenced by intersecting and multifactorial risk and resilience factors, and hence supports a psychosocial model when working with young people to better understand their mental health needs. This is in contrast to a biological, diagnostic approach which has limited value in adolescence, especially in the primary care setting.

Once the health practitioner has set the scene and put the young person at ease, the next step is to start to explore their presenting problems in a systematic and sensitive way; recognising that there may well be hidden or as yet unknown problems.

Globally the HEEADSSS tool is widely accepted, offering a comprehensive approach (see Table 7.1). It needs to be undertaken in steps and paced appropriately. This allows the young person to share issues which really matter to them. It helps build a trusting relationship with the family doctor, normalising the interaction.

Goldenring and Rosen devised the first version of this tool with the acronym HEADS (Home, Education & Employment, Activities, Drugs, Sexuality). They extended and updated it to the current version in 2004.[9] Sometimes, additional 'S''s are included, for Sleep and Spirituality.

It is important to emphasise that completion of the HEEADSSS tool should never be seen as mandatory and it is unlikely to be completed in the first consultation. A heavy-handed approach will negatively impact on the creation of a trusting therapeutic relationship and may result in the young person feeling rushed into discussing very personal information which has previously not been shared. HEEADASSS is best considered as an *aide memoire* and a guide to a thorough series of consultations.

**Table 7.1** The HEEADSSS Assessment Template

**Home and relationships**

- Who lives at home with you? Do you have your own room? Who do you get on with best/fight with most? Who do you turn to when you are feeling down?

**Education and employment**

- Are you in school/college at the moment? Which year are you in? What do you like the best/least at school/college? How are you doing at school? What do you want to do when you finish? Do you have friends at school? How do you get along with others at school? Do you work? How much? Is there a lot of pressure from home and/or school to achieve high grades? What is available if you leave school?

**Eating**

- Are you worried about your weight or body shape? Have you noticed any change in your weight recently? Have you been on a diet?

**Activities and hobbies**

- How do you spend your spare time? What do you do to relax? What kind of physical activities do you do? [At this stage – reassure about confidentiality]

**Drugs, alcohol and tobacco**

- Does anyone smoke at home? Lots of teenagers smoke. Have you been offered cigarettes? How many do you smoke each day? Include vaping. Many people start drinking alcohol as teenagers. Have you tried or been offered alcohol? How much/how often? Some young people use cannabis. Have you tried it? How much/how often? Include cannabis products, e.g. 'gummies', 'brownies'. What about other drugs, such as ecstasy and cocaine?

**Sex and relationships**

- Are you seeing anyone at the moment? Are they a boy or girl? Young people are often starting to develop intimate relationships. How have you handled that part of your relationship? Have you ever had sex? What contraception do you use?

**Self harm, depression and self image**

- How is life going in general? Are you worried about your weight? What do you do when you feel stressed? Do you ever feel sad and tearful? Have you ever felt so sad that life isn't worth living? Do you think about hurting or killing yourself? Have you ever tried to harm yourself?

**Safety and abuse**

- Do you feel safe at school/at home? Is anyone harming you? Is anyone making you do things that you don't want to? Have you ever felt unsafe when you are online or using your phone?

Source: adapted from Goldenring and Rosen, 2004

### 5. Scope out any possible risk areas.

As mentioned earlier young people may not know what is troubling them, or what lies at the root of their distress. It may lie in the immediate situation in which they find themselves or link back to earlier experiences which compromise resilience and increase vulnerability. It is important to undertake a developmentally and culturally appropriate risk assessment.

A 'good enough' primary care consultation will start to construct the building blocks of a therapeutically effective relationship whilst always be aware of co-existing risk factors. Carrying out a HEEADSSS conversation will reveal gaps in a young person's support network, financial problems, loneliness or pursuit of risky activities.

Identify who are the young person's supporting family members. Is their home environment safe? Are there any concerns about bullying, exploitation (criminal, sexual), abuse or neglect? Are they at risk because of behaviours related to drugs, alcohol or sex?

Are there additional vulnerabilities? Consider if the young person:

- Is a looked after child (fostered or adopted);
- has disabilities or long term health conditions;
- is an asylum seeker or refugee;
- is a young carer;
- has a minority sexual or gender identity (LGBTQ+).

A good risk assessment involves being able to understand whether the young person is emotionally mature enough to talk alone with the GP. Remember young people raised in an authoritarian household will struggle to speak autonomously at first and need gentle encouragement. Regarding their emotional maturity it may be helpful to follow the Fraser Guidelines and Gillick Competence, both established in the UK, while taking into account legal and moral standards in your own country.

The Fraser Guidelines[10] state that it is reasonable for a family doctor to provide contraception to a young person without parental consent if, in the doctor's opinion:

- the young person will understand the professional's advice;
- the young person cannot be persuaded to inform their parents;
- the young person is likely to begin, or to continue having, sexual intercourse with or without contraceptive treatment;

- unless the young person receives contraceptive treatment, their physical or mental health, or both, are likely to suffer;
- the young person's best interests require them to receive contraceptive advice or treatment with or without parental consent.

Gillick Competence is interpreted more broadly, to cover young people's consent to any medical intervention. According to the English lawyer Lord Scarman,

> As a matter of Law the parental right to determine whether or not their minor child below the age of sixteen will have medical treatment terminates if and when the child achieves sufficient understanding and intelligence to understand fully what is proposed.[11]

In summary, identifying Red Flags for a young person's safety must include identifying any immediate risk or threat to their personal safety, from a physical or online threat.

If any risks are identified, document and code them as your health recording system permits. You also need to be able to access clear local protocols about what to do if you are concerned. If you have a Safeguarding Lead, do you know who they are and how to contact them? Look out for local Updates and Continuing Professional Development opportunities in your area as this is a changing landscape and as professionals we often play 'catch-up' learning about challenges young people are already experiencing.

### 6. Undertake an appropriate physical examination.

You should be able to undertake a sensitive and developmentally appropriate examination. This would usually include:

- Height and weight;
- Outward behaviour including eye contact;
- Evidence of agitation or retardation of movement, restlessness;
- Evidence of self neglect;
- Evidence of pressure or slowness of speech.

### 7. Offer basic psychoeducation.

Depending on the problems the young person has presented, you should consider discussing one or more of these topics with them:

- Sleep;
- Exercise;

- Food intake and eating patterns;
- Substance use/abuse;
- Importance of healthy social relationships, both face-to-face and online;
- Social media use.

### 8. Offer simple relaxation techniques and strategies for de-stressing.

The information and advice presented in Chapter 3, on non-drug interventions, is as relevant to young people as it is to older adults. In addition to this, you can usefully scope out and recommend youth-friendly online resources which are available and accessible in your country. A good example from the UK is www.youngminds.org.uk.

### 9. Signpost for support.

As well as online resources, it is valuable for family doctors to get to know which local agencies providing youth-friendly care, and then to recommend these to young people in need.

### 10. Agree a follow-up plan.

Agreeing a follow-up plan is critical to closing the consultation safely. Arranging to meet again (or not, if it is agreed that there is no clinical indication to book an immediate follow-up appointment) demonstrates to the young person that they have been taken seriously, and that their worries and concerns are a legitimate use of clinician–patient time.

Always check up-to-date contact details, confirming their best contact telephone number and address. Check whether they are happy for mail to be sent to their home address. Seek consent to contact the young person if they miss a follow-up appointment. Set an alert in your system if possible.

## Service delivery

'State of the art' premises are desirable, but may be more feasible with private health providers than in cash-restricted public health sectors. For most young people, who are seeking help at a difficult time in their lives, the opportunity to speak with a kind, compassionate and thoughtful practitioner who is mindful of the developmental stages of adolescence is beneficial.

Health care practitioners need to be able to access professional training which supports their own development. Service leads, both clinical and managerial, need to invest in their staff and provide in-house training for 'front of house' personnel to provide the most appropriate and youth-friendly care they can offer.

The reception and waiting area are the first spaces young people will traverse before speaking with a health practitioner. Do they take into account young people as a population group whose needs are distinct and different from adults? Is it possible to make the reception and waiting area less intimidating and 'coldly clinical'? Are there posters and leaflets which acknowledge children and young people and their particular interests and needs? Posters in the waiting areas which clearly state how confidentiality is dealt with are key to building trust.

A key component to good service delivery is for local health care professionals to work with local youth service providers, both in the statutory and voluntary services. This might be achieved by informal meetings or more organised events at which all parties can become more familiar with each other's work. Young Ambassadors can be encouraged to work in health settings in a voluntary capacity or as part of a patient participation group.

Once good local relationships have developed, the act of signposting young people to local services becomes more meaningful. Family doctors become better able to address young people's fears of speaking, yet again, to another professional. Communication oils the wheels for young people to access local services more effectively.

Evaluation of service provision remains a key element of being assured that a health facility is respectful of young people's needs. For this to be undertaken effectively, young people should be involved as co-evaluators.[8]

# Educational material

### Case study

Kyle, aged 15, attends with his mother who tells you he is increasingly angry. He is getting into trouble with other members of the family, his teachers at school and has been cautioned by a police officer for shouting in a local park.

*What should you do next?*

- Advise his mother, and Kyle, that he needs to control himself or else he will get into even more serious trouble.
- Start a conversation with both initially, then with Kyle alone, beginning to explore what is happening for him.

Acting in an authoritarian manner without having any background knowledge will alienate Kyle and is likely to make the situation even more difficult for him and his mother. It is likely to mean that he would never consider talking to a health practitioner about how he is feeling in the future. So do not start by advising him to control himself.

Consultations with young people need to be rooted in the particular personal circumstances of their lives. Their behaviour and expressed emotions are directly related to the young person's specific context, both in the present and what has happened in the past.

You might want to consider what is already known about this young man's life from the consultation record, your own working knowledge of the family and the local community.

You offer time to the parent and Kyle, acknowledging that life must be a struggle at the moment, suggesting the parent has a chance to share what is worrying her, and then asking permission to the young man to speak with him alone whilst his mother waits outside.

You ask kindly, in an age appropriate manner, remembering young people do not have the same lexicon of words as an adult and when feeling distressed will have even less command of their language, what is happening for him in his life at the moment.

- Has there been any recent loss, bereavement or separation?
- Is there anyone at home or close to him who is seriously ill, or involved in a traumatic situation?

Try and start to build a picture of his immediate setting – who he lives with and if those adults in his life are able/in a position to address his basic needs of shelter, warmth, food and his emotional needs of being cared for, respected and kept safe.

Kyle tells you:

- His grandmother has died; he has lost contact with his dad; the family is breaking up.

- He has been smoking lots of cannabis, and with no income is getting into debt and resorting to petty crime.
- He views school as oppressive and his teachers uninterested in him as an individual.

*What is his main problem?*
- Loss of attachment.
- Drug addiction.

Drug use is common amongst young people in the community where you work. You know that for many youths it is a stage of their development to experiment with drug taking, drinking alcohol to excess and pushing boundaries of expected social norms and behaviours.

However, when it happens against a background of feeling unsupported, a strong sense of loss and without a trusted adult holding them in mind, drugs can fill a vacuum and numb painful emotions. Therefore, loss of attachment is his main problem.

*What is the best management plan?*
- Refer him to a local drug charity.
- Arrange to meet regularly to co-construct a plan.

Young people find it difficult to articulate what it is they need. Society does not treat them as equals to adults, and they are often unsure themselves what it is they are looking for. Therefore, meeting with him regularly is the best thing you can do at this stage.

Clarifying if Kyle is at risk from a family member or from someone outside of the home is essential; although it may not emerge in the first consultation. He will need to know he can trust you, and as with any human relationship trust needs time to build.

Your risk assessment will need to include whether he is self harming, for example, through punching walls or provoking fights, or in making risky decisions which might compromise his safety. Both in the present and every time you meet, it is important to review how things are progressing.

Over the next few consultations you aim to build up a trusting relationship, identify positive elements in Kyle's life and help him to describe his goals. Map your solution-focused approach to the local offers of youth provision; ideally encouraging Kyle to access effective outlets for frustration, such as sport or music.

# Multiple choice questions

For family doctors working with young people:

1. Which of these elements of the working environment is *unlikely* to be helpful?

   a. A clean and comfortable reception area.
   b. A long wait for an appointment.
   c. Youth-friendly posters.
   d. Privacy in the consultation.

2. When would you not consider breaking confidentiality?

   a If the young person is doing something their parents would disapprove of.
   b If the young person is at risk of harming themselves.
   c If the young person is at risk of harming someone else.
   d If the young person is at risk of being harmed by someone else.

3. Which of these topics is *not* included in a HEEADSSS assessment?

   a. Home and relationships.
   b. Education and employment.
   c. Respiratory function tests.
   d. Self harm and abuse.

4. It may be reasonable to provide contraception to a young person without parental consent if:

   a. The young person cannot understand the professional's advice.
   b. The young person can be persuaded to inform their parents.
   c. The young person is unlikely to begin, or to continue having, sexual intercourse with or without contraceptive treatment.
   d. Unless the young person receives contraceptive treatment, their physical or mental health, or both, are likely to suffer.

5. When arranging a follow-up appointment with a young person, which of the following is *not* good practice?

a. Check up-to-date contact details, including telephone number.
b. Check whether they are happy for mail to be sent to their home address.
c. Seek consent to contact them if they miss the follow-up appointment.
d. Inform their parents if they miss a follow-up appointment.

You will find the answers to these MCQs on page 171.

# Resources

A valuable touchstone exists in the WHO document: *Making health services adolescent friendly: developing national quality standards for adolescent friendly health services* (2012) which serves as a practical guide:

www.who.int/maternal_child_adolescent/documents/adolescent_friendly_services/en/

Many countries have developed their own variations. For example, in 2016 the Department of Health in the UK produced a gold standard check list – *'You're Welcome'* – for health care settings to review provision of youth-friendly health care:

www.youngpeopleshealth.org.uk/yourewelcome/
Other useful resources include:

1. WHO. Health for the world's adolescents: a second chance in the second decade: www.who.int/maternal_child_adolescent/documents/second-decade/en/
2. Lancet Standing Commission on Adolescent Health & Well-being: www.adolescentsourfuture.com
3. NHS England. *15 Steps Challenge: Children and Young People's Toolkit*: www.england.nhs.uk/wp-content/uploads/2018/06/15-Steps-30-May.pdf
4. Association for Young People's Health: *GP Champions for Youth Health Project*: www.youngpeopleshealth.org.uk/wp-content/uploads/2015/06/GPToolkit_ONLINE.pdf
5. Paul Hamlyn Foundation. *Right Here: How to Provide Youth Friendly Mental Health Services.* www.phf.org.uk/publications/improve-mental-wellbeing-youth-work-practice/

International LGBT Association: www.ilga.org

# References

1. Sawyer S, Afifi R, Bearinger L, et al. Adolescence: a foundation for future health. *Lancet.* 2012, 379: 1630–1639.
2. Kieling C, Baker-Henningham H, Belfer M, et al. Child and adolescent mental health worldwide: evidence for action. *Lancet.* 2011, 378: 1515–1525.
3. Patel V, Flisher AJ, Hetrick S, McGorry P. Mental health of young people: a global public-health challenge. *Lancet.* 2007, 369: 1302–1313.
4. Youth access. Young people in mind. London, 2014. www.youthaccess.org.uk/down loads/ypimtheyoungpeople.pdf [accessed 29 April 2019].
5. Morgan C, Webb RT, Carr MJ, et al. Incidence, clinical management, and mortality risk following self harm among children and adolescents: cohort study in primary care. *BMJ.* 2017, 359: j4351.
6. Patton GC, Sawyer SM, et al. Our future: a Lancet commission on adolescent health and wellbeing. *Lancet.* 2016, 387: 2423–2478.
7. Roberts Jane H, Crosland A, Fulton J. 'I think this is maybe our Achilles heel ...': exploring GPs' responses to young people presenting with emotional distress in general practice: a qualitative study. *BMJ.* 2013, 3: e002927.
8. Tylee A, Haller DM, Graham T, et al. Youth-friendly primary-care services: how are we doing and what more needs to be done? *Lancet.* 2007, 369: 1565–1573.
9. Goldenring J, Rosen D. Getting into adolescent heads: an essential update. *Contemporary Pediatrics.* 2004, 21: 64.
10. Cornock M. 'Fraser guidelines or Gillick competence?' *J Child Young People Nursing.* 2007, 1: 142.
11. UK House of Lords Decisions [AC 112]. www.bailii.org/uk/cases/UKHL/1985/7.html [accessed 29 April 2019].

# Chapter 8

# FRAILTY AND MULTIMORBIDITY

Christos Lionis and Marientina Gotsis

# Key points

1. Assessment tools and the initial contact with family doctors.
2. Informing the patient and meeting the patient's family.
3. Planning for patient support: the interface with the primary care team.
4. Monitoring the patient with frailty: clinical tools.
5. The clinical management of frailty.
6. Innovation in care with traditional and emerging tools.
7. Towards integrated care for patients with frailty.
8. Issues for future research.

# Introduction

Multimorbidity and frailty are two concepts that, when both co-exist, are known to lead to increased falls, caregiver dependency, hospitalization, disability, and mortality.[1-4] Much interest has been placed recently on the relationship between measured frailty and mental health/psychiatric illness: they can be considered as mutual risk factors (the one can lead to the other), and some reviews have shown a positive association between the two conditions.[5,6] However, the cause and effect cycles are often unclear. This discussion has led to an important question: to what extent are frailty and depression separate constructs, different manifestations of the same under-lying entity, or related causative factors? The current area of research interests includes the variation of frailty across cultures, the creation of risk prediction models based on frailty status, and the identification of potentially modifiable risk factors associated with frailty, psychological wellbeing, and intervention.[7] Of particular interest is the emerging concept of cognitive frailty.[8]

Current literature discusses interventions with potential impact to decrease or prevent long term adverse outcomes, such as falls, disability, and premature death. Other major issues include the relative benefits and risks of psychoactive medications in those with significant co-morbidities and frailty: for example, the moderating role of newer generation antidepressants remains unclear. While late-age depression and frailty share several pathophysiologic mechanisms, including subclinical cerebrovascular disease, inflammation, and dysregulation of the hypothalamic-pituitary-adrenal axis,[9] the ultimate goal is the design of effective interventions to reduce the burden and improve outcomes among individuals and families affected by frailty and mental health disorders; and some of these may be nonmedical in action. Although primary care (PC) seems to be a suitable setting for effectively managing this patient population, the condition is frequently under-diagnosed. The severe effects on both quality of life and cost of health care services make this an important area of research and practice.

Both concepts, frailty and multimorbidity, are contested terms. For the individual, it is possible to have multiple diagnoses: some patients with Type 2 diabetes, hypertension, and musculoskeletal disorders still feel healthy and have good quality of life, while others have very poor health and quality of life. This raises questions regarding the incidence and frailty phenotype association only with ages 65 years and over since frailty can also affect younger people.[10-13] Given that precursors of frailty tend to arise earlier in the life-course,[13] there is increased importance for early recognition of pre-frailty and prevention of its progression to the frailty phenotype.[1]

For carers, the term of frailty suggests a situation that is serious and irreversible, while for clinicians the term is not always "top of mind".[14] There is no widely accepted consensus on frailty. An operational definition has been published by Fried et al. as follows: "Frailty is characterized by a loss of functionality leading to an increased vulnerability to adverse stress and health events."[1] Similarly, McDonagh et al. defined frailty as a multidimensional syndrome characterized by a state of increased vulnerability to acute stressors, such as hospitalization, falls and infection.[15] In a current position paper, experts agreed on the importance of a more comprehensive definition of frailty that should include assessment of physical performance, including gait speed and mobility, nutritional status, mental health, and cognition.[16] In addition, an interesting concept that has recently received attention is that of cognitive frailty.[8,17]

Frailty is a known concept in the UK, and some GPs are paid to manage such cases as part of Local Enhanced Service (LES) contracts.[18] However, it is still unknown in certain primary care settings and patients and families are not typically involved in its discussion. It is important to understand how patients and others experience frailty from a phenomenological perspective.

Susan Pickard explains "during the experience of bodily disruption that leads to felt frailty, bodily movements become foregrounded, impeding bodily motility ... 'taken-for-granted' skills have to be relevant, as well as new ones acquired."[19] She introduces the concept of "being 'out of place' in one's familiar surroundings" as a commonly felt experience among elderly who had experienced falls. Participants in various studies described the experience as "a complete reversal of my life", "intolerable", "defeated", and one where the subject was seen as a universal "symbol of frailty". For some, things are even worse: Caroline Nicholson et al. describe this phase as a "drawn out, uncertain and dwindling process of dying."[20] The psychosocial and existential dimensions of frailty underscore the necessity of compassion, creativity, and collaboration between individual, social environment, and health professionals.

It is critical to underline the impact of frailty and relevant associated multimorbidity on family medicine. On a practical level, it involves patients and families from different clinical disciplines and health-related specialties, including cardiologists, psychologists, social workers, neurologists, physical therapists, oncologists, and internists. It creates a huge need for integration and coordination between general practitioners/family physicians (GPs/FPs, hereafter referred to as "Family Doctors" (FDs)). In general, the purpose of addressing these clinical entities is not to involve medical disciplines, but also to invite the interdisciplinary team to work with the individuals and family at the community level. The discussion opens an additional door for collaboration with non-health professionals in the realm of arts and technologies, a relatively new domain for general practice/family medicine.

Frailty seems to be a suitable subject for an integrative and holistic approach that is well tailored with the definition of family medicine,[21] and could be used as a clinical case to read, translate, and interpret the recently approved WHO Declaration on Primary Health Care made in Astana.[22] Also, frailty is a multi-component clinical entity that includes the cognitive, physical, and mental domains. This complexity requires interventions not only toward the patients, but also for their family, and their communities in general. It implies the necessity of communication and clinical skills – diagnostic, therapeutic, and rehabilitative. The interface of the FD with the patient who progressively declines emotionally and physically, or with a family member who is affected by this growing burden, underscores the value of this wider scope for practical guidelines aimed at FDs.

The implications of frailty on the delivery of services are another issue that has not always received the attention it deserves. The burden to the formal care services, the risks of associated polypharmacy, and the major impact of frailty and multimorbidity on family health and resources all need recognition and action. The complex nature of multi-domain interventions for frailty has some evidence that points to improved outcomes, compared to mono-domain (single level) intervention,[23-25] with early cost-comparisons showing some benefit for very frail community-dwelling individuals compared to usual care.[25] In general, interventions for frailty are more effective when they focus on discoverable deficiencies, when they are theory-driven if client-centred, and when they offer group-based social motivation.[24]

This chapter addresses frailty and multimorbidity as key concepts in PC clinical practice and research with a main focus on frailty, its multiple components, tools for its assessment and monitoring, and its effective management.

# Service delivery

Frailty and its associated multimorbidity call for integrated care services that offer a suitable clinical setting to deliver effective, well organized, coordinated, and comprehensive primary health care. Before this, we must identify the patients where such approaches are needed. So here we address the tools that can be used for early diagnosis of frailty, for planning the initial contact with family, and for the tasks assigned to the FD and primary care team regarding care services – as well as sharing guidelines for referral to community-based support and rehabilitation services.

### 1. Assessment tools and the initial contact with FDs

A key question for FDs is who should receive screening for frailty. There is no consensus on this, but screening for frailty phenotype is recommended for the following conditions:

People aged 60 plus years:

a. with a worsening chronic health condition, including heart failure, cancer, dementia, musculoskeletal disability, and chronic neurological and psychiatric diseases; or

b. with significant multimorbidity, i.e. five or more illnesses and chronic conditions and polypharmacy; or

c. after admission and an extended stay in hospital or after a major surgical operation.

A recent publication from the UK suggests that "Efforts to identify, manage, and prevent frailty should include middle-aged individuals with multimorbidity, in whom frailty is significantly associated with mortality, even after adjustment for number of long term conditions, sociodemographics, and lifestyle."[10]

Another question is: "What tools are suitable for screening in primary care?" There are many papers in the literature that address this subject. Some of them report assessment tools based on the findings of a systematic review, while others discuss selected tools. The scope of the different reviews varies: some look at tools relevant to patients with cardiovascular disease[26] or with a more specified disease or age group[27] like heart failure, while there are also published papers that discuss frailty under the scope of family doctors.[28] The literature is also rich with papers making recommendations for frailty assessment tools that address some specific areas or domains of assessment including slowness, weakness, low physical activity, exhaustion, and shrinking.[9,27] National Health Services in England[14] defined five major domains on which to perform a comprehensive geriatric assessment: medical, mental health, functional capacity, social circumstances, and environment.

To begin screening for frailty and identify the "frailty phenotype", FDs have at their disposal questionnaires such as the Simple Frail Scale,[29] the Simplified Fried test,[1] the Short Physical Performance Battery (SPPB),[30] the 5m Gait Speed,[31] and the PRISMA 7.[32]

The Simple Frail Scale is easy to implement and does not require any instruments. The Fried criteria tool requires the use of one dynamometer. The Gait speed test – average speed to walk meters[31] – is recommended in primary care. Based on a systematic review by Harrison et al.,[33] the slow gait speed, PRISMA 7, and the timed get-up-and-go test have high sensitivity for identifying frailty: however, limited specificity implies many false-positive results, which means that these instruments cannot be used as accurate single tests to identify frailty.

## 2. Informing the patient and meeting the patient's family

Informing the patient about diagnosis and prognosis is always an important task for FDs. Informing a patient about the diagnosis of frailty is not an easy job. Frailty is not a disease but a status that indicates that the patient's capacity to react to normal stressors has declined. It is a complicated status with many manifestations across various systems and functions that enhance the probability of hospital admission and potential death. Pre-frailty and early stages of frailty are potentially reversible, but it depends on the underlying causes and the associated multimorbidity.

However, FDs should make the patient and their family aware of the severity of the situation, as well as the support that is required to avoid possible hospital admission and high cost. A family conference is recommended at this point. It could be arranged either at the doctor's office or at home, depending on patient status.

The completion of some selected tools, including the Groningen Frailty Indicator,[34] the Edmonton Frail Scale,[35] and the Frailty Staging System[36] offer the chance to have a discussion jointly with the family members about issues of integrated care, functionality, and daily activities. Comprehensive Geriatric Assessment (CGA)[37] is also recommended as an evaluation method of the elderly person's psychosocial, medical, functional, and environmental issues. The Geriatric Depression Scale[38] is included in the current CGA. Other instruments that can include assessment of depression and psychological functioning are the Deficit Accumulation Index[39] and the Tilburg Frailty Indicator.[40]

Assessment needs to reflect the skills and capacity of practitioners in the primary care team. The linkage of this team with specialists is another issue that needs attention when effective care for people with frailty is considered.

### 3. Planning for the patient support: the interface with the primary care team

The role of the primary care team in supporting frailty and multimorbidity is widely recognized. There is an active discussion in the literature about the multiple components of frailty: cognitive, mental, physical, and nutritional.

### 4. Monitoring the patient with frailty: clinical tools

There are several domains of physical, mental, and spiritual health, as well as social and daily life that FDs should monitor after a diagnosis of frailty:

    a.  Functionality (including mobility);
    b.  Self-reported physical activity, exercise tolerance, and exhaustion;
    c.  Presence of symptoms (including appetite, memory loss (cognition), depressive feelings, sleep disorders);
    d.  Presence of signs (including weight loss);
    e.  Control of co-morbidities;
    f.  Review of medication adherence, and non-prescription intake.

Efforts should be made to monitor the progress of symptoms like exhaustion, loss of appetite, and others that denote depression. The identification of mild cognitive impairment (MCI) is also important since MCI and frailty frequently coexist leading researchers to make assumptions like this that "these entities are unequivocal prodromal stages of a future disease."[8] The role of FDs in motivating individuals with frailty to participate in the therapeutic plan is very significant at this stage.

## 5. The clinical management of frailty

Currently, there is a debate on the effectiveness of the various interventions to meet the needs of patients with frailty. There is no official consensus about the effectiveness of specific actions and interventions aiming to alter the natural course of frailty. However, the roles of FDs and the primary care team need to serve two important goals:

    a. To reduce symptoms that frequently relate to underlying conditions and morbidities (i.e. symptoms related to angina, heart failure, arrhythmias, cancer, dementia, depression).

    b. To reduce the risk of complications or adverse outcomes.

The following interventions can achieve this:

- Paying attention to the risk of complications from medical procedures (less-invasive strategies are preferred);
- Avoiding complications resulting from inappropriate prescribing and overdosing;
- Reducing the risk of falls and the incidence of fragile structure;
- Arranging a shorter stay in hospital and offering long term support after any discharge.

The 2013 consensus by Morley et al.[29] suggests four domains of intervention for the clinical management of frailty especially related to exercise, dietary counselling, and polypharmacy.

There is consistent evidence about the benefit of exercise-related interventions in aging,[41] although there is not much evidence in relation to mental illness and older adults, except in depression.[42,43] However a limited literature search which attempted to respond to the research question "What is the effectiveness of exercise interventions to reverse or delay the progression of frailty in those with frailty?" reported that there is sufficient evidence that shows the effectiveness of exercise interventions to reverse or delay the progression of frailty in those with frailty.[44] FDs should be trained in advising about and supervising aerobic and resistance programmes jointly with physiotherapists and the primary care team,[45] although more evidence from future research is required.[7] Resistance exercises build muscle strength and tone, as well as bone, which can reduce falls in older people. There is also much discussion on the role of dietary counselling. A dietary plan that provides 25–30g of high-quality protein per meal under the form of a nutritional supplement has been recommended to prevent muscle mass loss. Prescribing other nutritional supplements for the patient with frailty, such as vitamin D and calcium, is still under debate with unresolved controversies.

Another goal for FDs when they manage patients with frailty is to reduce unnecessary medications for both cost-savings and adverse effects. The implementation of Beers criteria has been recommended.[46] The Screening Tool of Older Persons Prescriptions and Screening Tools to Alert Treatment criteria have also been recommended by a recent review.[33]

FDs should also manage the frequently co-existing mental health disorders including that of depression. The two "overlapping" syndromes of frailty and depression in late life have already been mentioned. Major depression is not rare in older adults and it can be treated with antidepressants and electroconvulsive therapy. However, in mild to moderate depression, psychological therapies and exercise are recommended. We have discussed these in Chapter 3. In cases where an antidepressant may be effective, outcomes depend on polypharmacy and what other drugs patients are on, but antidepressants tend to present a high risk for adverse events.[47]

## 6. Innovation in care with traditional and emerging tools

Promising interventions that are arts and/or technology-driven with a frailty focus are in early trials,[48] from screening tools of cognitive function[49] to digital arts-based physical therapy,[50] game-console-based exergaming,[51,52] and even virtual agents to address loneliness.[53] Virtual reality is an especially powerful technology that could be used more in the future for assessment,[54] and for neurorehabilitation that combines cognitive-motor outcomes.[55] Although it is exciting to think about new technologies in the future, it is crucial to address the innovative aspects of care delivery from the standpoint of human-centered "experience design". This means that we must first look to the more established art forms of creative and multi-sensory engagement with patients, especially in settings where technology will not easily penetrate for years and decades to come. The benefits of arts and media-based interventions do not lie in the material aspect of delivery (analog vs. digital), but in the overall experience, which can be evidence-based or practice-based.

Art therapy has a long history in health care[56–58] and can help address the multi-dimensional aspects of frailty from physical strength to existential woes. For example, positive outcomes have been measured with dance-based interventions for prevention of worsening of frailty outcomes,[59] for behavioral issues and mood improvement in dementia,[60] and for balance improvement in older adults in general.[61] Palliative care has a long tradition of using art therapy to help address aspects of identity, control, grief, and community.[56] Improvement of cognitive-motor benefits are not so relevant in palliative care but there is a general under-standing that embodied arts and kinaesthetic involvement can address issues of self and mind in a more holistic manner.[56] Play and interactive entertainment-based interventions using games have also been explored with a focus on frailty showing improvements across physical fitness, executive function, and emotional regulation outcomes.[62] Robert et al. document the challenges and opportunities in this future area of media and technology with pragmatism, including addressing ethical challenges, and the unresolved technological literacy deficits and related biases in the health professions.[61]

Lastly, there is room for improvement in interventions related to frailty if we take into consideration the research in multisensory environ-ments. One must appreciate the overall environmental factors on the built and natural environment that can have a significant impact on daily life, in a health care setting, and in community-dwelling.[63,64] Studies show that addressing light, texture, color, sound and noise, and interior and exterior architectural elements can directly affect frailty and related physiological, emotional, economic, service-use-related, sleep, engagement, behavioral and psychological, cognition-related, and function-related outcomes.[64]

The Department of Health Service and Population Health at King's College London is working on the creation of risk prediction models based on frailty status to understand likely outcomes that the individual may face.[7]

## 7. Towards integrated care for patients with frailty

The World Health Assembly defines integrated health services as:

> health services that are managed and delivered so that people receive a continuum of health promotion, disease prevention, diagnosis, treatment, disease management, rehabilitation and palliative care services, coordinated across the different levels and sites of care within and beyond the health sector and according to their needs throughout the life course.[65]

The use of clinical entities like frailty to guide the design and refinement of new educational curricula incorporating integrated, patient-centered, and compassionate care may also facilitate the understanding of necessary actions towards change, and health care reform. The integration of primary health (PH) into primary health care (PHC) could be a first step to initiate the discussion about integrated care in several European settings. It could facilitate the implementation of the second stem that will link primary care with mental, hospital, and social care. Training and empowering patients, families, caregivers, health professionals, and policymakers to define and promote integrated care could motivate an important step in that direction.

Two hot issues in the effective management of patients with heart failure are discharge planning and specialist follow-up. The latest guidelines of the European Society of Cardiology on heart failure[66] recommend that all patients who are discharged from the hospital should be reviewed by their GPs within one week and by a hospital cardiology team within two weeks of discharge.

ADVANTAGE Joint Action is a work co-funded by the European Union and 22 Members States to develop a common European approach to the prevention and management of frailty. In one of its perspective papers, Hendry et al.[67] suggest a model of care that would incorporate the following:

- A single entry point in the community (most likely primary care);
- The use of simple frailty-specific screening tools across care settings;
- Comprehensive assessment and individualized care plans that are inclusive of caregivers;
- Tailored interventions by interdisciplinary teams, both in hospitals and in the community;
- Shared electronic information tools, and technology-enabled care solutions.

## 8. Issues for future research

As reported above, the Department of Health Service and Population at King's College London is working on the creation of risk prediction models based on frailty status to understand likely outcomes faced by individuals. Part of the undertaken research focuses on anxiety and depression as important contributors to frailty. In addition, research on risk prediction models may assist both clinicians and policymakers.[7]

# Educational material

## Case study

An 85-year-old woman with heart failure, mixed type of dementia, hypertension, dyslipidemia, and atrial fibrillation, lives in a nursing home. She is very much dependent on personal aids for daily living. The institution's carers assist her but there is no specific mobilizing daily programme to support her. She remembers some people and past events, expresses several emotions, and asks to return to her home.

*What is her main problem?*
- To what extent has her multimorbidity contributed to her current status?
- Can you identify any mental health disorders?

*What should you do next?*
- Could you manage her main problems without team assistance?
- Can you identify their main tasks?

*What is the best management plan?*
- How can you best meet and manage her physical, mental, cognitive, and social care problems?

# Multiple choice questions

1. Which of the following health conditions could lead to frailty?

   a. Dementia.
   b. Anaemia.
   c. Heart failure.
   d. COPD.
   e. Cancer.
   f. All the above.
   g. a, c, d and e.

2. Select two of the following treatment choices to meet the needs of a person with frailty.

   a. Vitamin D.
   b. Dietary supplements.

    c. Daily resistance exercises.

    d. Motivational interviewing in combination with cognitive behavioral therapy.

    e. Vitamins complex A and B.

3. Which two of these therapeutic strategies are least appropriate for the aforementioned clinical case of the 85-year-old woman in her current state?

    a. Expressive arts therapy.

    b. Horse therapy.

    c. Individual psychotherapy.

    d. Group dance.

    e. Sensory stimulation.

You will find the answers to these MCQs on page 171.

## Further reading and e-resources

Frailty. Net Resource Portal
http://frailty.net/

Waterloo Wellington Integrated Health Programs eLearning Modules on Frailty
www.regionalhealthprogramsww.com/frailtymodules/#frailty

British Geriatrics Society – Frailty Resources
www.bgs.org.uk/topics/frailty

Life Circles – Brief documentary film of a dance project with the frail elderly
https://vimeo.com/40647427

Healing Spaces – Brief documentary film of a multisensory interactive experience for older adults with advanced dementia
https://vimeo.com/271410883

The Elder Project (2010) – Documentary film about seven seniors experiencing frailty over the course of two years
www.nfb.ca/film/elder_project/

## References

1. Fried LP, Tangen CM, Walston J, et al. Frailty in older adults: evidence for a phenotype. *J Gerontol Series A* 2001, 56(3): M146–M157.
2. Speechley M, Tinetti M. Falls and injuries in frail and vigorous community elderly persons. *J Am Geriatr Soc* 1991, 39(1): 46–52.

3. Winograd CH. Targeting strategies: an overview of criteria and outcomes. *J Am Geriatr Soc* 1991, 39(S1): 25S–35S.

4. Boeckxstaens P, Vaes B, Legrand D, et al. The relationship of multimorbidity with disability and frailty in the oldest patients: a cross-sectional analysis of three measures of multimorbidity in the BELFRAIL cohort. *Eur J Gen Practice* 2015, 21(1): 39–44.

5. Buigues C, Padilla-Sánchez C, Garrido JF, et al. The relationship between depression and frailty syndrome: a systematic review. *Aging & Mental Health* 2015, 19(9): 762–772.

6. Cherry S, Peel N, Hubbard R. The relationship between measured frailty and psychiatric illness: a systematic review. *PROSPERO* 2016. Available from: https://www.crd.york.ac. uk/prospero/display_record.php?ID=CRD42016033678. CRD42016033678.

7. UK Research and Innovation: Health Service and Population Research. Exploring frailty, mental health and related outcomes: a multi-cultural population-based approach to ageing. https://gtr.ukri.org/projects?ref=MR/K021907/1 [Accessed: 21st April 2019].

8. Canevelli M, Cesari M. Cognitive frailty: far from clinical and research adoption. *JAMA* 2017, 18(10): 816–818.

9. Vaughan L, Goveas J, Corbin A. Depression and frailty in later life: a systematic review. *ClinI Interven Aging* 2015, 10: 1947.

10. Hanlon P, Nicholl BI, Jani BD, et al. Frailty and pre-frailty in middle-aged and older adults and its association with multimorbidity and mortality: a prospective analysis of 493 737 UK Biobank participants. *Lancet Pub Health* 2018, 3(7): e323–e332.

11. Theou O, Rockwood MRH, Mitnitski A, Rockwood K. Disability and co-morbidity in relation to frailty: how much do they overlap? *Arch Gerontol Geriat* 2012, 55(2): e1–e8.

12. Rockwood K, Song X, Mitnitski A. Changes in relative fitness and frailty across the adult lifespan: evidence from the Canadian National Population Health Survey. *CMAJ* 2011, 183(8): E487–E494.

13. Mitnitski A, Rockwood K. The rate of aging: the rate of deficit accumulation does not change over the adult life span. *Biogerontol* 2016, 17(1): 199–204.

14. NHS England. Frailty resources. www.england.nhs.uk/ourwork/clinical-policy/older-people/frailty/frailty-resources/ [Accessed: 21st April 2019].

15. McDonagh J, Martin L, Ferguson C, et al. Frailty assessment instruments in heart failure: a systematic review. *Eur J Cardiovas Nursing* 2018, 17(1): 23–35.

16. Rodríguez-Mañas L, Féart C, Mann G, et al. Searching for an operational definition of frailty: a Delphi method based consensus statement. *J Gerontol Series A* 2013, 68(1): 62–67.

17. Feng L, Zin Nyunt MS, Gao Q, et al. Cognitive frailty and adverse health outcomes: findings from the Singapore Longitudinal Ageing Studies. *JAMA* 2017, 18(3): 252–258.

18. Fit for frailty | British Geriatrics Society. www.bgs.org.uk/resources/resource-series/fit-for-frailty [Accessed: 7th July 2019].

19. Pickard S. Health, illness and frailty in old age: a phenomenological exploration. *J Aging Stud* 2018, 47: 24–31.

20. Nicholson C, Meyer J, Flatley M, et al. Living on the margin: understanding the experience of living and dying with frailty in old age. *Soc Sci Med* 2012, 75(8): 1426–1432.

21. Lionis C, Petelos E, Papadakis S, et al. Towards evidence-informed integration of public health and primary health care: experiences from Crete. *WHO Public Health Panorama* 2018, 4(4): 491–735.

22. Declaration on Primary Health Care 2018. [Online] World Health Organization (WHO). Available from: www.who.int/primary-health/conference-phc/declaration [Accessed: 4th May 2019].

23. Dedeyne L, Deschodt M, Verschueren S, et al. Effects of multi-domain interventions in (pre)frail elderly on frailty, functional, and cognitive status: a systematic review. *Clin Intervent Aging* 2017, 12: 873–896.

24. Gwyther H, Bobrowicz-Campos E, Apóstolo J, et al. A realist review to understand the efficacy and outcomes of interventions designed to minimise, reverse or prevent the progression of frailty. *Health Psychol Rev* 2018, 12(4): 382–404.

25. Apóstolo J, Cooke R, Bobrowicz-Campos E, et al. Effectiveness of interventions to prevent pre-frailty and frailty progression in older adults. *JBI Database System Rev* 2018, 16(1): 140–232.

26. Singh M, Stewart R, White H. Importance of frailty in patients with cardiovascular disease. *Eur Heart J* 2014, 35(26): 1726–1731.

27. Afilalo J, Alexander KP, Mack MJ, et al. Frailty assessment in the cardiovascular care of older adults. *J Am Col Cardiol* 2014, 63(8): 747–762.

28. Lionis C, Midlöv P. Prevention in the elderly: a necessary priority for general practitioners. *Eur J Gen Practice* 2017, 23(1): 203–208.

29. Morley JE, Vellas B, Abellan van Kan G, Anker SD, Bauer JM, Bernabei R, et al. Frailty consensus: a call to action. *J Am Med Dir Assoc* [Online] Elsevier; 2013, 14(6): 392–397. doi:10.1016/J.JAMDA.2013.03.022 [Accessed: 22nd April 2019].

30. Guralnik JM, Ferrucci L, Simonsick EM, et al. Lower-extremity function in persons over the age of 70 years as a predictor of subsequent disability. *NEJM* 1995, 332(9): 556–562.

31. van Kan G, Rolland Y, Andrieu S, Bauer J, Beauchet O, Bonnefoy M, et al. Gait speed at usual pace as a predictor of adverse outcomes in community-dwelling older people: an International Academy on Nutrition and Aging (IANA) Task Force. *J Nutr Health & Aging* [Online] 2009, 13(10): 881–889. Available from: www.ncbi.nlm.nih.gov/pubmed/19924348 [Accessed: 5th May 2019].

32. Hebert R, Raiche M, Dubois M-F, et al. Impact of PRISMA, a coordination-type integrated service delivery system for frail older people in Quebec (Canada): a quasi-experimental study. *J Gerontology Series B* 2010, 65B(1): 107–118.

33. Harrison JK, Clegg A, Conroy SP, et al. Managing frailty as a long-term condition. *Age Ageing* 2015, 44(5): 732–735.

34. Peters LL, Boter H, Buskens E, Slaets JPJ. Measurement properties of the Groningen Frailty Indicator in home-dwelling and institutionalized elderly people. *JAMA* 2012, 13(6): 546–551.

35. Rolfson DB, Majumdar SR, Tsuyuki RT, et al. Validity and reliability of the Edmonton Frail Scale. *Age Ageing* 2006, 35(5): 526–529.

36. Lachs MS, Feinstein AR, Cooney LM, et al. A simple procedure for general screening for functional disability in elderly patients. *Ann Int Med* 1990, 112(9): 699–706.

37. Welsh TJ, Gordon AL, Gladman JR. Comprehensive geriatric assessment: a guide for the non-specialist. *Int J Clinical Practice* 2014, 68(3): 290–293.

38. Hoyl MT, Alessi CA, Harker JO, et al. Development and testing of a five-item version of the geriatric depression scale. *J Am Geriatr Soc* 1999, 47(7): 873–878.

39. Cohen HJ, Smith D, Sun C-L, et al. Frailty as determined by a comprehensive geriatric assessment-derived deficit-accumulation index in older patients with cancer who receive chemotherapy. *Cancer* 2016, 122(24): 3865–3872.

40. Gobbens RJJ, van Assen MALM, Luijkx KG, et al. The Tilburg Frailty Indicator: psychometric properties. *JAMA* 2010, 11(5): 344–355.

41. Rebelo-Marques A, De Sousa Lages A, Andrade R, et al. Aging hallmarks: the benefits of physical exercise. *Frontiers Endocrinol* 2018, 9.1–15.

42. Catalan-Matamoros D, Gomez-Conesa A, Stubbs B, et al. Exercise improves depressive symptoms in older adults: an umbrella review of systematic reviews and meta-analyses. *Psychiatr Res* 2016, 244: 202–209.

43. Rhyner KT, Watts A. Exercise and depressive symptoms in older adults: a systematic meta-analytic review. *J Aging Physical Activity* 2016, 24(2): 234–246.

44. Gray C, Argáez C. Exercise interventions for the delayed progression or reversal of frailty 2018. https://cadth.ca/exercise-interventions-delayed-progression-or-reversal-frailty [Accessed: 9th July 2019].

45. Aguirre LE, Villareal DT. *Physical Exercise as Therapy for Frailty* 83. Nestle Nutrition Institute workshop series, 83–92. 2015.

46. Beers Criteria Medication List - DCRI. https://dcri.org/beers-criteria-medication-list/ [Accessed: 22nd April 2019].

47. Kok RM, Reynolds CF. Management of depression in older adults. *JAMA* 2017, 317(20): 2114.

48. Fanfarelli JR. Games and dementia: evidence needed. In: Ferguson CJ (ed.) *Video Game Influences on Aggression, Cognition, and Attention*. Cham: Springer International Publishing, 2018. 163–171.

49. Silva Neto H, Cerejeira J, Roque L. Cognitive screening of older adults using serious games: an empirical study. *Entertainment Computing* 2018, 28: 11–20.

50. Gardner P, Surlin S, McArthur C. ABLE: an arts-based, interactive physical therapy platform for seniors with dementia and frailty. In: Stephanidis C (ed.) *HCI International 2018*. Cham: Springer International Publishing, 2018. 140–148.

51. Gomes GCV, Bacha JMR, do Socorro Simões M, et al. Feasibility, safety, acceptability, and functional outcomes of playing Nintendo Wii Fit Plus™ for frail elderly: study protocol for a feasibility trial. *Pilot and Feasibility Studies* 2017, 3(1): 1–7.

52. Fu AS, Gao KL, Tung AK, et al. Effectiveness of exergaming training in reducing risk and incidence of falls in frail older adults with a history of falls. *Arch Physical Med Rehab* 2015, 96(12): 2096–2102.

53. Sidner CL, Bickmore T, Nooraie B, et al. Creating new technologies for companionable agents to support isolated older adults. *ACM Transactions Interactive Intelligent Systems* 2018, 8(3): 1–27.

54. Coughlan G, Coutrot A, Khondoker M, et al. Toward personalized cognitive diagnostics of at-genetic-risk Alzheimer's disease. *Proc Nat Acad Sci* 2019, 116(19): 9285–9292.

55. Serino S, Barello S, Miraglia F, et al. Virtual reality as a potential tool to face frailty challenges. *Frontiers Psychol* 2017, 8: 8–11.

56. Beilharz K, Poulos C, Poulos R, et al. *Creative Art Making in Palliative Care*. Textbook of Palliative Care. London: Routledge, 2018. 1–21.

57. Jones DP. *The Arts Therapies*. London: Routledge, 2004.

58. Eickholt J, Geretsegger M, Gold C. Perspectives on research and clinical practice in music therapy for older people with depression. In: Zubala A, Karkou V (eds.) *Arts Therapies in the Treatment of Depression*. Oxon, UK: Routledge, 2018. 227–254.

59. Machacova K, Vankova H, Volicer L, et al. Dance as prevention of late life functional decline among nursing home residents. *J Applied Gerontol* 2017, 36(12): 1453–1470.

60. Guzmán A, Freeston M, Rochester L, et al. Psychomotor Dance Therapy Intervention (DANCIN) for people with dementia in care homes: a multiple-baseline single-case study. *Int Psychogeriatr* 2016, 28(10): 1695–1715.

61. Robert PH, König A, Amieva H, et al. Recommendations for the use of serious games in people with Alzheimer's disease, related disorders and frailty. *Frontiers Aging Neurosci* 2014, 6: 1–13.

62. Filar-Mierzwa K, Długosz M, Marchewka A, et al. The effect of dance therapy on the balance of women over 60 years of age: the influence of dance therapy for the elderly. *J Women Aging* 2017, 29(4): 348–355.

63. Bowes A, Dawson A. *Designing Environments for People with Dementia*. 2019, Published online: 18th Jan 2019. Permanent link to this document: https://doi.org/10.1108/978-1-78769-971-720191004. 1–92.

64. Silva R, Abrunheiro S, Cardoso D, et al. Effectiveness of multisensory stimulation in managing neuropsychiatric symptoms in older adults with major neurocognitive disorder. *JBI Database Syst Rev* 2018, 16(8): 1663–1708.

65. WHO global strategy on people-centred and integrated health services. WHO. 2015. www.who.int/servicedeliverysafety/areas/people-centred-care/global-strategy/en/ [Accessed: 22nd April 2019].

66. Ponikowski P, Voors AA, Anker SD, et al. ESC guidelines for the diagnosis and treatment of acute and chronic heart failure. *Eur Journal Heart Failure* 2016, 18(8): 891–975.

67. Hendry A, Carriazo AM, Vanhecke E, et al. Integrated Care: a Collaborative ADVANTAGE for Frailty. *Int J Integrated Care* 2018, 18: 2.

Chapter 9

# MANAGING PATIENTS WITH DEMENTIA

Ferdinando Petrazzuoli, Christos Lionis and Venetia Young

# Key points

1. Dementia is a clinical syndrome with several causes which creates impairments in mental ability, personality, affect and socialisation.
2. Information from family members can be very useful in the early identification of cognitive impairment.
3. Patients presenting with cognitive impairment should be evaluated for potentially reversible causes, with a range of laboratory tests and investigations.
4. Sharing the diagnosis is one of the hardest parts of dementia care. Family doctors (FDs) should give information gradually and sensitively.
5. Dementia medications have only modest efficacy. It is encouraged to discuss the risks, side effects and benefits with the patient and family.
6. Non-pharmacological management such as regular structured routine, good sleep hygiene, reminiscence and cognitive stimulation can help to improve the wellbeing of patients with dementia.
7. During the course of dementia most patients develop behavioural and psychological symptoms of dementia (BPSD). These result in a lower quality of life, high caregiver burden and psychotropic drug use.
8. When the burden of care exceeds the resources of the caregiver, nursing home placement commonly ensues.
9. When patients with dementia lack mental capacity to make decisions about areas of their lives, legal processes may be necessary.
10. In dementia care there are considerable differences between countries and within countries.

# What is dementia?

Dementia is a clinical syndrome with several causes, which leads to a variety of disabilities: cognitive, emotional (depression, anxiety, agitation) and physical.[1] The introduction of the term neurocognitive disorder attempts to help reduce the stigma associated with the word dementia. Patients may prefer the term "ageing brain" and the concept of brain failure. Major neurocognitive disorder is a decline in mental ability severe enough to interfere with independence and activities of daily living.

**Types of dementia**

- Alzheimer's disease
- Vascular dementia
- Mixed Alzheimer's and vascular dementia
- Lewy body dementia (LBD)
- Fronto-temporal dementia
- Huntingdon's disease
- Multiple sclerosis
- Alcoholic dementia

The different dementias have different patterns of presentation and pathways of deterioration. Prescribing needs may vary with each type. Alzheimer's disease is slowly progressive. Vascular dementia may show a stepwise deterioration. Lewy body dementia may present with visual hallucinations and fronto-temporal dementia with personality changes and disorders of executive function.

Mild cognitive impairment (MCI) is a popular definition for mild neurocognitive disorder. MCI is a common condition in the elderly with a prevalence of 16.0% in individuals without dementia and an incidence rate of 63.6 (per 1,000 person-years).

*MCI differs from dementia in that it is not severe enough to interfere with independence in daily life.*

In a German study the weighted total prevalence of MCI was 20.3%, while in the Cretan Aging Cohort, which comprised 3140 persons aged ≥ 60 years living in a rural area, the prevalence of MCI was much higher (32.4%).[2]

**Early detection of mild cognitive disorder**

Early identification of cognitive impairment would ideally allow patients and their families to receive care at an earlier stage in the disease process, which could lead to improved prognosis and decreased morbidity. Health, psychological, and social benefits from early recognition of dementia through education and improved decision making may make screening valuable, even if early treatment cannot alter the natural history of dementia by preventing or slowing the rate of cognitive decline.

There are several arguments against case finding and increasing the number of diagnoses of MCI: prognostic uncertainty; a risk of false positive diagnoses; the risk of stigmatisation, social isolation, losing perspective with suicidal ideation; the lack of an effective cure for dementia.

**Relevance of the problem**
*According to the Alzheimer Report 2015 it is estimated that 46.8 million people worldwide were living with dementia in 2015.*

It is predicted that this number will almost double every 20 years, reaching 75 million in 2030 and 131 million in 2050.[3]

# Recognising the symptoms and signs of dementia in the primary care setting

Early identification and management of dementia in the primary care setting continues to be challenging. Common early symptoms of dementia include:

- Memory problems, particularly for recent events;
- Increasing confusion;
- Reduced concentration;
- Personality or behaviour changes;
- Apathy and withdrawal;
- Depression and loss of ability to do everyday tasks.

Before using the classical dementia tools (Mini Mental State Evaluation (MMSE), Clock Drawing test) and starting a formal evaluation, consider using a short questionnaire with a close relative (Figure 9.1). One of these is the informant interview included in "The General Practitioner assessment of Cognition (GPCOG)".

**Informant interview questions**
- Does the patient have more trouble remembering things that have happened recently than s/he used to? Does s/he have more trouble recalling conversations a few days later?
- When speaking, does the patient have more difficulty in finding the right words or tend to use the wrong words more often?
- Is the patient less able to manage money and financial affairs (e.g. paying bills, budgeting)?
- Is the patient less able to manage his or her medication independently?
- Does the patient need more assistance with transport (either private or public)? (If the patient has difficulties due only to physical problems, e.g. bad leg, tick "no".)

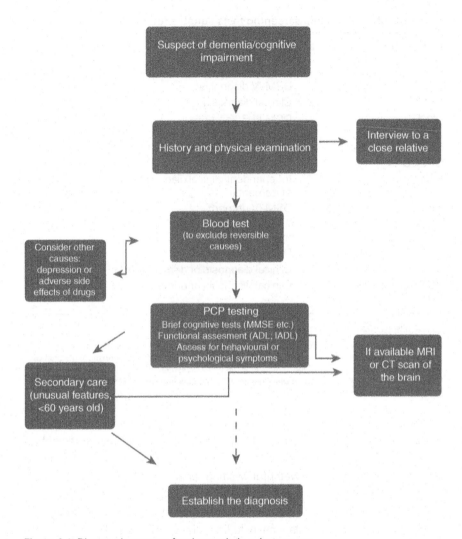

**Figure 9.1** Diagnostic process for dementia in primary care

### What preliminary tests have a value for family doctors?

There are plenty of tools for the establishment of the possibility of dementia. Table 9.1 is a list of some short tests suitable for primary care.[4,5]

*FDs should use brief dementia specific screening tests, master one or two and use them frequently. No test has definitively proved to be better than the others.*

MMSE is the most popular test in several primary care settings, but with some exceptions, e.g. the United Kingdom where the copyright is an

**Table 9.1** Short dementia screening tests suitable for primary care

| Instrument | Time to use (min) | Gold standard | Cut-off |
|---|---|---|---|
| MMSE | 5–10 | DSM-IV diagnosis | 23/24 |
| AMTS | 3–4 | Clinical diagnosis | 6/7 |
| Clock-Drawing test | 3 | DSM III-R dementia | Schulman method, Score 2/3 |
| 6-CIT | 3–4 | Clinical diagnosis of dementia | 7/8 |
| GPCOG | 6 | DSM-IV dementia | 10/11 on total score |
| Mini-Cog | 3 | Independent clinical diagnosis of dementia | Probably normal/ possibly impaired |
| TYM | 5–10 | DSM-IV dementia | 30/31 |
| MoCA | 10 | Clinical diagnosis of Alzheimer's disease | 25/26 |
| ACE-R | 15–20 | DSM-IV dementia | 73/74 |
| MIS | Under 5 | Clinical diagnosis of dementia | 5/6 |
| AQT Color-Form | Under 5 | Clinical diagnosis of dementia | 70.5 seconds |

Source: adapted from Sheehan et al. 2012[6]

6-CIT: Six Item Cognitive Impairment Test; ACE-R: Addenbrookes Cognitive Assessment-Revised; AMTS: Abbreviated Mental Test Score; AQT: A Quick Test of Cognitive Speed; DSM: Diagnostic and Statistical Manual of Mental Disorders; GPCOG: General Practitioners Assessment of Cognition; Mini-Cog: Mini-Cog Screening for Cognitive Impairment in Older Adults; MIS: Memory Impairment Screen; MMSE: Mini-Mental State Examination; MoCA: Montreal Cognitive Assessment; TYM: Test your Memory.

increasingly pressing issue and where newer dementia tools are becoming more popular.[7,8] In most cases this preliminary evaluation is sufficient to optimise referral to a secondary care specialist. In other cases it may be preferable to employ a watchful waiting approach. Depending on local protocols, the FD involvement in the dementia diagnostic workup can vary from country to country. It is important that these tests can be used with all kinds of primary care populations including rural populations. The GPCog and TYM have proved to be reliable tools also in rural settings.[4]

FDs should also consider tests to assess the functional abilities of older people. Activities of daily living (ADLs) include the skills typically needed to manage basic physical needs: bathing, dressing, toileting. These functional skills are mastered early in life and are relatively more preserved in light of declined cognitive functioning compared to higher level tasks. Instrumental activities of daily living (IADLs) include more complex activities related to independent living in the community (shopping, food preparation, managing finances and medications). IADL impairment can often present in early dementia, whereas basic ADL declines are often not present until later stages of dementia.

**The diagnosis of dementia in low and middle income countries (LMICs)**

The diagnosis of dementia in LMICs can be particularly challenging for a variety of reasons: the lack of sophisticated techniques of neuroimaging, the low educational level of the population, cultural prevailing beliefs about mental illness and the scarcity of dementia tools scientifically validated in this particular setting. The paucity of specialised physicians on this topic and the exiguity of a coordinated and integrated health care system add to the problems.

The probability that symptoms really reflect cognitive problems increases with time, and we do need to establish a diagnosis as early as possible. We could start with a simple motivational technique to enhance rapport and engagement and we should exclude some secondary causes of dementia with simple lab tests. We need to make sure that all we do respects the person's wishes, expectation and values including those related to his/her culture and religion or spiritual beliefs.

We may use a variety of laboratory tests to help diagnose dementia and/or rule out other conditions. A basic list includes a complete blood count, Vitamin B12 level, blood glucose test, urinalysis, drug and alcohol tests (toxicology screen), and thyroid-stimulating hormone levels.[9] Tests for certain infections known to cause dementia, such as HIV and syphilis, and other tests may be ordered as appropriate according to the probability of this condition affecting the patient in his/her local setting.

Not all the tools for dementia have proved to be acceptable and suitable in LMICs. Some tests which seem effective in these settings are the TYM, GPCOG and the AQT. FDs should also assess the functional abilities of older people and in particular the ADLs, which include the skills typically needed to manage basic physical needs, and in the case of MCI, the IADLs or a similar test culturally adapted.

In LMICs, physicians are invited to address a few questions to the close relatives during the interviewing either at the beginning (of the engagement) or later on.

As stated in another part of this guidance, a good relationship with the family and the patients themselves is essential. It is important to use a locally and culturally adapted style of conversation with the patients and their families. As a general rule, the patient with the disease should never be excluded from conversations. Responding to patient and caregiver emotions and fostering a sense of hope and meaning should therefore be the preferred approach. Above all, we should all bear in mind the message which McDaniel et al. have reported in their book, "Family Oriented Primary Care",[10] i.e. the necessity of:

- giving guidance to the family about the capacity of the health care system;
- coordinating the patient's care with a multidisciplinary team;
- advocating for the family and the patient to keep their autonomy;
- consulting them in their decision-making;
- collaborating with the caregivers and supporting both family and caregivers.

## Identifying modifiable cognitive impairment

Patients presenting with cognitive symptoms should be evaluated with a range of laboratory tests, ECG and with structural brain imaging (computed tomography (CT) or magnetic resonance imaging (MRI)), if available in their setting.

Other tests include:

- Full blood screen;
- ESR, CRP (inflammatory markers);
- Blood glucose;
- Kidney and liver function;
- Thyroid function;
- Vitamin B12;
- Syphilis and HIV;
- Calcium.

Potentially reversible cognitive impairment should be identified, and treatment considered, even if partial or full reversal of the cognitive symptoms cannot be guaranteed. The most frequently observed potentially reversible conditions identified in patients with cognitive impairment or dementia are:

- Medication, especially any drug with anticholinergic activity;
- Depression;
- Delirium;
- Metabolic (hypothyroid);
- Hypo or hypercalcaemia;
- Diabetes;
- Normal pressure hydrocephalus;
- Tumour or subdural haematoma;
- Infection (syphilis, HIV/AIDS);
- Anaemia (vitamin B12 or folate deficiency);
- Alcohol abuse;
- Vision and hearing declining.

Depression is the most recognisable potentially reversible condition, and it is also a risk factor for dementia. Delirium is also common. It occurs alongside infections and other illnesses and may resolve a long time after discharge. People with dementia are more susceptible to delirium.

**Dementia and multimorbidity**

There is a high prevalence of comorbidity in older people with dementia, especially cardiovascular diseases and depression. Individuals with depression or severe depressive symptoms experience faster cognitive decline over time.[11,12] We have discussed this in more detail in Chapter 8.

*Middle aged and older populations are increasingly taking multiple drugs, with potential adverse events of long-term use.*

Anticholinergic drugs are used for depression, hypertension, gastrointestinal disorders, Parkinson's disease, lower urinary tract dysfunction (LUTS), epilepsy, and to manage allergies. Anticholinergics affect cognition and guidelines suggest they are to be avoided among frail older people as it is advisable to use alterative drugs (Table 9.2). Above all it is the vascular

**Table 9.2** Anticholinergics and other drugs to be used with caution in dementia

| Medication | Avoid | Use |
|---|---|---|
| Bladder instability | Tolteridone Oxybutinin | Solifenacin |
| Antiemetics | Cyclizine Metochlopramide Prochlorperazine | Domperidone Ondansetron |
| Antihistamines | Chlorpheniramine Promethazine Hydroxyzine | Loratadine Fexofenadine |
| Analgesics | Tramadol Pethidine | Paracetamol |
| Tricyclics | Avoid – including Amitriptyline | |
| Sedation Benzos | Diazepam Nitrazepam Temazepam Zopiclone | Lorazepam prn only Chlormethiazole |
| Antidepressants and Anxiolytics | Citalopram | Sertraline Trazodone Mirtazepine 15mg |
| Antipsychotics | Haloperidol (except in delirium) Avoid all in dementia in Parkinson's disease and Lewy body dementia | Risperidone Quetiapine For short periods and low doses |

and metabolic comorbidities along with frailty which are more frequently associated with dementia.

# Reducing the risk of dementia

Most of the risk factors for dementia are exactly the same as those for cardiovascular diseases: type 2 diabetes, smoking, hypertension, obesity, physical inactivity. This fact enhances the role and the impact of FDs when they assess patients with multimorbidity and a high cardiovascular risk; and so FDs are certainly expected to endorse the "Healthy Brains in Healthy Hearts" approach.[12,13] Living alone increases by 50% the risk of developing dementia. FDs should suggest that elderly patients avoid this isolation. Participation in physical leisure activities can reduce the risk of dementia in subjects with MCI. Physical exercise also has a positive effect on preventing falls in older adults with cognitive impairment. The traditional Mediterranean diet delays cognitive decline.

Secondary prevention consists of cognitive rehabilitation therapies in an attempt to slow the decline in cognitive and functional performance; patients need to remain involved in the intervention until a therapeutic effect can be attained.

# Disclosing the diagnosis

Diagnostic disclosure is the first step in the process of adjustment to dementia as a neurological long-term condition, both for the people with dementia and their caregivers. When disclosing the diagnosis, the best way involves:

- Preparing;
- Exploring patient perspectives;
- Involving the family;
- Sharing the diagnosis;
- Communicating effectively;
- Responding to patient reactions;
- Focusing on quality of life;
- Planning for the future.

If family members wish to shield the patient from the diagnosis, the FD should find out the underlying concerns; in most cases disclosure to the patient is the best approach. Fostering a sense of hope and meaning is essential.

## Service delivery

Once the diagnosis is established there are many encouraging actions which are included in the post-diagnostic phase (Figure 9.2).

### Specialist referral
In many countries the role of the FD is limited in the respect of dementia. This is particularly true in countries where a specific preauthorisation by a secondary care specialist is essential in order to have the dementia medication reimbursed by the local health care system.[7] A preliminary

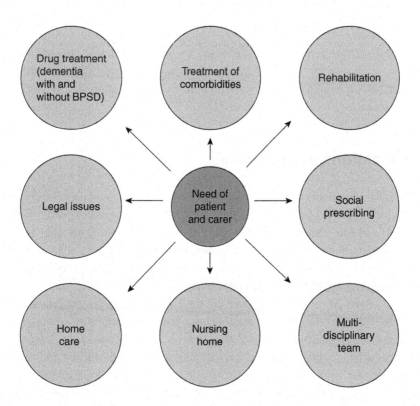

**Figure 9.2** Dementia: post-diagnostic support

primary care dementia diagnosis workup is very useful to carefully select the patients to refer to secondary care specialists.

### Teams and integrated approaches in the community

The priority is to understand what the patient and family need at each stage along the dementia illness journey. They need to know who is available to be called in to help. Establishing a multidisciplinary team (MDT) is highly advisable. This team could include:

- Geriatric psychiatrist;
- Geriatrician;
- Psychiatric nurse;
- Clinical psychologist;
- Medical social worker;
- Occupational therapist;
- Physiotherapist;
- Speech and language therapist;
- Neurologist

Care should be provided by the team with a named lead clinician who takes responsibility for the whole process of care.[14] There may be charitable organisations that can provide volunteer support for patients and carers.

# Medications in dementia

Cognitive enhancers are two types of medications: acetylcholinesterase inhibitors and N Methyl-D-aspartate (NMDA) receptor antagonists (Table 9.3). These may be beneficial for patients with Alzheimer's disease, producing slowing or stabilisation of the illness, improving memory, behaviour and activities of daily living. They produce modest therapeutic benefits by regulating neurotransmitter function to maintain cognitive function.

Because of the concerns on their efficacy, some countries have adopted completely different approaches. The High Authority of Health in France has decided that the anti-Alzheimer drugs no longer have a place in the therapeutic strategy (lack of clinical relevance of the efficacy and risk of side effects) and will not reimburse them anymore. In the UK, NICE guidance promotes dual therapy: acetylcholinesterase inhibitors plus

**Table 9.3** Characteristics and side effects of medication for dementia

| Drug | Dose | Common side effects | Comments |
|---|---|---|---|
| **Acetylcholinesterase inhibitors** | | | |
| Donepezil | Start with 5 mg, increase to 10 mg after ≥ 4 wk | Oral medicines: nausea, vomiting, diarrhoea, bradycardia | |
| Rivastigmine capsule | 1.5 mg BD, titrate to 6 mg BD | | • Contraindicated in bradycardia; exercise caution in peptic ulcer disease |
| Rivastigmine patch (transdermal) | Rivastigmine Patch 5, increase to Patch 10 after ≥ 4 wk | Skin patch: rash, itch; fewer gastrointestinal side effects | • Donepezil: some brands are orodispersible. A generic version of donepezil is now available |
| Galantamine | The tablets and liquid are to be taken twice a day, preferably with morning and evening meals. The extended-release capsules are usually taken once a day in the morning. Dosage to be increased gradually, maximum recommended dose of 24 milligrams per day | Nausea, vomiting, stomach pain, diarrhoea, dizziness, loss of appetite, weight loss, tiredness, bradycardia, irregular heartbeat, fainting, and seizures | • For gastrointestinal side effects, stop for a week, then restart; some patients may tolerate the drugs on rechallenging |
| **NMDA receptor antagonist** | | | |
| Memantine | 5–20 mg daily (titrate from 5 mg) | Headache, giddiness; constipation at higher doses; rarely paradoxical insomnia | • Approved for moderate to severe Alzheimer's disease; can be used as monotherapy or in combination with donepezil • If creatinine clearance < 30 mL/min, max 10 mg daily |

memantine after a single drug is no longer effective. This is in line with the latest Cochrane Library Review (March 2019) on memantine:

> clinical heterogeneity in AD makes it unlikely that any single drug will have a large effect size, and means that the optimal drug treatment may involve multiple

drugs, each having an effect size that may be less than the minimum clinically important difference.[15]

The clinician should aim to optimise the patient's chronic disease management to decrease the risk of a cardiovascular event.

## Behavioural and psychological symptoms of dementia (BPSD)

In the case of severe BPSD a specialist consultation is essential. It is important to minimise the use of atypical antipsychotics as they increase the stroke risk. During the course of dementia most patients develop some types of neuropsychiatric symptoms, with a lower quality of life, high caregiver burden, psychotropic drug use and a major risk of institutionalisation.

Severe BPSD symptoms which may lead to institutionalisation include:[16]

- Delusions;
- Wandering;
- Agitation;
- Apathy;
- Hallucinations;
- Paranoia;
- Aggression;
- Aberrant motor behaviour;
- Anxiety;
- Irritability;
- Disinhibition;
- Sleep disturbance;
- Suicidal ideation.

## Non-pharmacological management of dementia
### *Non-pharmacological interventions should be the first-line management.*

In severe cases, non-pharmacological intervention still has a valuable adjunctive role with pharmacological treatment.[17] With ongoing follow-up FDs/nurses should think about: dentition, oral thrush, swallowing and diet, bowel and bladder function, joint pain and mobility, ear wax, vision, Vitamin D deficiency and regular medication review.

## Communication with a patient affected by dementia

The communication skills of a person with dementia will gradually decline as the disease progresses. The disease affects each person differently. Tips for successful communication are suggested by the Alzheimer's Association (www.alz.org/).

- Do not exclude the person with the disease from conversations;
- Speak directly to the person rather than to his or her caregiver or companion;
- Take time to listen to the person express their thoughts, feelings and needs;
- Give the person time to respond;
- Do not interrupt unless help is requested.

Structured daily activities, including regular gentle exercise and cognitive activities, help patients with dementia to maintain mental function. Insomnia is common and often distressing to families. Good sleep hygiene helps both dementia patients and their caregivers to have more energy to face their daytime demands. Caffeine should be avoided.[17]

## Reminiscence and other activities

Reminiscing activities can help seniors with dementia feel contented and peaceful, enhance positive feelings, improve mood, reduce agitation and minimise challenging behaviours such as wandering.

Cognitive stimulation (CS) is one of the most popular non-pharmacological interventions which has proved to have some positive effect in dementia. It is based on a range of enjoyable activities providing general stimulation for thinking, concentration and memory and it is administered usually in a small group. Several studies report that CS may delay functional impairments and improve quality of life (QoL) in people with dementia.

## Cognitive impairment-related safety issues

Safety issues such as wandering out of the house, getting lost or forgetting to switch off the gas can be risky for both patients and their families.

*Safety issues for patients and their families*
- Electric cooker instead of a gas cooker;
- Use appliances that can turn off automatically;
- Smoke and carbon monoxide detector installation;

- Medication locked away;
- Keep all cleaning products secured.

## Supporting family and other caregivers

The caregiver burden can be defined as a multidimensional response to the negative appraisal and perceived stress resulting from taking care of an ill individual. It threatens the physical, psychological, emotional and functional health of the caregiver.[18]

*Caregiver burden and burnout should be identified promptly by primary care physicians.*

A useful tool to evaluate the caregiver burden is the Involvement Evaluation Questionnaire-European Union (IEQ-EU).[19] More educational awareness and support from the community would help to relieve some of the stress and prevent caregiver burnout.

## Intermediate care

*Intermediate care is an excellent method of supporting the caregiver.*

Intermediate care is defined as health care occurring between traditional primary (community) and secondary (hospital) care settings. High quality intermediate care is important and may prevent caregiver burnout.

Listed below are various examples of intermediate care.

- Integrated at-home services;
- Respite/relief services;
- Day care centres;
- Nursing and residential homes.

## Admission to a nursing home

People with dementia are generally cared for in their community by family members for a large portion of the duration of their illness. However, when the burden of care exceeds the resources of the caregiver or causes deficits in the life of the caregiver, nursing home placement commonly ensues.

The decision to place a relative in a nursing home can be complex, long, and agonising for family caregivers, and is frequently delayed as long as possible in response to caregivers' feelings of responsibility and guilt.

*In many societies sending a person to a nursing home is still considered unfilial. FDs should choose the best way to raise this point as the family caregiver may feel diminished by this suggestion.*

Key to a successful and effective nursing home placement for primary family caregivers of persons with dementia is the support for their decision and advice from staff, FDs, health care workers, family and friends.[17]

The relationship to the person with dementia seems to influence reasons for institutionalisation along with the presence of neuropsychiatric symptoms.

*In countries where nursing homes are not so common, a strong familial network seems to be an effective substitute.*

### Community support for people with dementia

*FDs should play an active role working on the key determinants of active and healthy ageing.*

In order to tackle the care of old frail people with dementia in an effective way, health and social care services need to be integrated and need to offer prevention programmes that will help older adults stay connected to the social world, so that they can continue to experience well-being despite physical incapacities and maintain a sense of self-esteem.

One of the best approaches to support people with dementia and their caregiver is "Social Prescribing", which can be defined as a mechanism for linking patients with non-clinical sources of support within the community. It also helps to bring communities together and break down social isolation. Engaging patients in arts, social activities and interacting within their communities makes them feel more involved, more confident and more resilient. Relationships are a basic human need.

# Legal issues for dementia sufferers and families

There are many legal issues which emerge as a person with dementia ages: will, power of attorney, advance life decisions, surrendering of driving licence.

*FDs should check that legal issues are being dealt with by the family.*

It can be helpful to get consent for information sharing when the patient is relatively well, as this can make end of life care more straight-forward. Ideally everyone will have made their end of life wishes clear.

Issues become more complex if there are elements of abuse occurring. Then safeguarding processes may have to be implemented.

Although elder abuse can take many forms, there is broad agreement that the following are among the most significant:

- Physical abuse;
- Sexual abuse;
- Psychological/emotional abuse;
- Financial or economic abuse;
- Neglect and acts of omission;
- Racial/discriminatory abuse;
- Domestic abuse;
- Institutional abuse.

FDs need to be clear about their reporting lines for these incidents.

There may be situations where patient choice may be at odds with the view of the FD and it becomes a challenge to manage respect for patient autonomy with the desire to prevent avoidable harms.

*In the absence of serious crime, and of significant risks to third parties, competent adults retain the right to make decisions about how they wish to direct their lives.*

In the UK, the Mental Capacity Act 2005 (MCA) provides the legal definition of capacity; it is a guide on how to assess whether someone has the capacity to make a situation specific decision and provides the legal framework for acting and making decisions on behalf of individuals who lack the mental capacity to make particular decisions for themselves.

*Doctors should presume that adults have the capacity to consent to or refuse a proposed treatment unless it can be established that they lack that capacity.*

It may be appropriate to involve the local Adult Social Care institutions, or the psychiatry team if mental health problems or neurological deficits appear to be impacting on the patient's capacity and if the family are in disagreement.

## Lasting powers of attorney (LPA)
In the UK, individuals who have mental capacity can appoint an attorney under an LPA, to make financial, health and welfare decisions on their behalf once they lose capacity.

*Unless it is an emergency, consent from the attorney is required for all decisions that would have required consent from the adult had he/she retained capacity.*

# End of life

*Given the choice, most people would prefer to die in their own homes, and with appropriate support more families could be enabled to care at home until the end of life.*

At present, in Western societies, people with dementia often die outside the family home. In other societies dying at home is still common but often it represents an additional burden for the family caregiver.

FDs should be aware that the "home" represents a feeling of familiarity, comfort and security and is associated with the concept of a "good death". Atul Gawande's five questions for end of life care may still be appropriate even with dementia.[20]

Unfortunately, many people receive suboptimal care at home and are admitted to hospital where they receive active treatment rather than palliative care and comfort measures. Admissions to nursing homes can cause confusion and resulting behavioural problems. However, as a person with dementia moves into the later stages of the disease, they typically need a more extensive level of care than their family can provide.

Signs of the terminal stage may be swallowing difficulties and concomitant chest infections, difficulty walking and speaking, and recurrent urinary tract infections. Attention to pain and how the patient expresses this, their hydration needs, and mouth care are important.

*Family caregivers commonly receive help from their children, other family members and siblings, as well as friends and neighbours, volunteers and religious acquaintances, and this is a great help especially in less developed countries.*

*In facilitating end of life care at home for people with dementia, GPs can help skilled informal caregivers to appropriately manage symptoms and administer medications to minimise distress.*

# Educational material

### Case study

Your patient is an 82-year-old woman. She is a widow with 12 children, and has always worked as a housewife. She lived alone until diagnosed with dementia. She has been on dementia drugs for two years (memantine) but without success. Her last MMSE score was 9. She has the following co-morbidities: cerebrovascular disease (aortic valve replacement, heart failure and atrial fibrillation), diabetes mellitus, hypertension, hyperlipidemia, glaucoma and osteoporosis.

She attends the consultation with her daughter. Her presenting problems are loss of appetite and weight, and a notable deterioration in her abilities. She can no longer cook safely, as she leaves the stove on. She does not recognise her relatives, and has insomnia.

*What are her main problems?*
- Progression of dementia and frailty;
- Weight loss;
- Family disagreements.

*What happened next?*
- Her family disagreed about her care. She had lived with her daughter for 18 months, but her daughter could no longer cope.
- She was referred to hospital. She had a long inpatient stay, during which a PEG tube was inserted. She died a few weeks after admission to nursing home.
- Her last year of life was undignified.

*What could have happened?*
- Her wishes for end of life care could have been ascertained when she was well and had mental capacity.
- Members of her family could have been appointed by her, to make decisions about finance and wellbeing in advance. If there were still disagreements, then social care might have advised further legal involvement.
- Mental capacity assessment and safeguarding processes could have been instigated, to protect her as a vulnerable adult at risk of family and iatrogenic harm.
- Referral to old-age psychiatry or a geriatrician with multiagency team, including a Speech and Language Therapist for swallowing assessment.
- Thorough physical assessment including checking for oral candidiasis, UTI and other easily treatable causes of weight loss (but probably not looking for cancer).
- Rationalisation of her medications.
- Team discussions in hospital to reach better decisions about her, involving her FD who had known her for a long time.

- Frank conversations with the family, over time, about the physical and mental frailty meaning that she was at the end of life. Giving them a plan for her to die with dignity.
- Assessment of the daughter's wellbeing and her need to share the burden.

*What is needed for the primary care team?*
Training in:

- End of life decision making;
- Mental capacity assessments;
- Challenging conversations in dementia;
- Carer assessments.

# Multiple choice questions

1. Which of the following is a core symptom of dementia?

   a. Dizziness.
   b. Memory problems.
   c. Fatigue and weakness.
   d. Neuropathic pain.

2. Which of the following diseases or conditions is often present in patients with dementia?

   a. Cardiovascular diseases.
   b. Depression.
   c. Anxiety.
   d. All of the above symptoms or diseases.

3. Which of the following drugs is *not* a typical drug for dementia?

   a. Memantine.
   b. Donepezil.
   c. Piracetam.
   d. Rivastigmine.

4. Which of the following statements is *not* true?

   a. Mild cognitive impairment always evolves into dementia.
   b. According to DSM-V mild cognitive impairment is called mild neurocognitive disorder.
   c. Mild cognitive impairment can be considered a transitional state between normal and pathologic cognitive decline.
   d. Individuals with major neurocognitive disorder exhibit cognitive deficits that interfere with independence, while persons with mild neurocognitive disorder may retain the ability to be independent.

You will find the answers to these MCQs on page 171.

# Further reading and e-resources

### Recommended books

Prince M, Wimo A, Guerchet M, et al. World Alzheimer report 2015: the global impact of dementia. Alzheimer's Disease International (ADI), London, 2015.

James O. *Contented dementia: 24-hour wraparound care for lifelong well-being.* Random House, 2008.

Gawande A. *Being mortal: medicine and what matters in the end.* Metropolitan Books, 2014.

### Useful websites

Understanding Dementia. Massive Open Online Course. University of Tasmania, Australia. https://mooc.utas.edu.au/courses/understanding-dementia-2019-02

National Institute of Clinical Excellence Pathways. Dementia overview. http://pathways.nice.org.uk/pathways/dementia

Dementia Pathways. PREPARED. Department of General Practice. University College Cork http://dementiapathways.ie/education

World Health Organization mhGAP Intervention Guide - Version 2.0 for mental, neurological and substance use disorders in non-specialised health settings

www.who.int/mental_health/mhgap/mhGAP_intervention_guide_02/en/

# References

1. Iliffe S, Manthorpe J. Dementia: is the biopsychosocial model vindicated? *Br J Gen Practice.* 2017, 67(661):344–345.
2. Zaganas IV, Simos P, Basta M, et al. The Cretan aging cohort: cohort description and burden of dementia and mild cognitive impairment. *Am J Alzheimer.* 2019, 34(1):23–33.
3. Prince M, Wimo A, Guerchet M, et al. World Alzheimer report 2015: the global impact of dementia. Alzheimer's Disease International. ADI, London, 2015.

4. Iatraki E, Simos PG, Bertsias A, et al. Cognitive screening tools for primary care settings: examining the 'test your memory' and 'general practitioner assessment of cognition' tools in a rural aging population in Greece. *Eur J Gen Practice*. 2017, 23(1):171–178.

5. Brodaty H, Low LF, Gibson L, Burns K. What is the best dementia screening instrument for general practitioners to use? *Am. J. Geriatr. Psychiatry*. 2006, 14(5):391–400.

6. Sheehan B. Assessment scales in dementia. *Ther. Adv. Neurol. Diso*. 2012 Nov, 5 (6):349–358.

7. Petrazzuoli F, Vinker S, Koskela TH, et al. Exploring dementia management attitudes in primary care: a key informant survey to primary care physicians in 25 European countries. *Int Psychogeriatr*. 2017, 29(9):1413–1423.

8. Creavin ST, Wisniewski S, Noel-Storr AH, et al. Mini-Mental State Examination (MMSE) for the detection of dementia in clinically unevaluated people aged 65 and over in community and primary care populations. *Cochrane Database Syst Rev*. 2016, (1): CD011145.

9. Adelman AM, Daly MP. Initial evaluation of the patient with suspected dementia. *Am Fam Physician*. 2005, 71(9):1745–1750.

10. McDaniel SH, Campbell TL, Hepworth J, Lorenz A. *Family-oriented primary care*. Berlin: Springer Science & Business Media, 2005 Dec 6.

11. Clague F, Mercer SW, McLean G, et al. Comorbidity and polypharmacy in people with dementia: insights from a large, population-based cross-sectional analysis of primary care data. *Age Ageing*. 2017, 46(1):33–39.

12. Lionis C, Midlov P. Prevention in the elderly: a necessary priority for general practitioners. *Eur J Gen Practice*. 2017, 23(1):202–207.

13. Livingston G, Sommerlad A, Orgeta V, et al. Dementia prevention, intervention, and care. *Lancet*. 2017, 390(10113):2673–2734.

14. Dowrick C. Patient-centred care for multimorbidity: an end in itself? *Lancet*. 2018, 392 (10141):4–5.

15. McShane R, Westby MJ, Roberts E, Minakaran N, Schneider L, Farrimond LE, Maayan N, Ware J, Debarros J. Memantine for dementia. Cochrane Database of Systematic Reviews. 2019, Issue 3. Art. No.: CD003154. DOI: 10.1002/14651858.CD003154.pub6

16. Brodaty H, Connors MH, Xu J, et al. The course of neuropsychiatric symptoms in dementia: a 3-year longitudinal study. *JAMA*. 2015, 16(5):380–387.

17. Poon NY, Ooi CH, How CH, Yoon PS. Dementia management: a brief overview for primary care clinicians. *Singapore Med J*. 2018, 59(6):295.

18. Schoenmakers B, Buntinx F, Delepeleire J. What is the role of the general practitioner towards the family caregiver of a community-dwelling demented relative? A systematic literature review. *Scand J Prim Health Care*. 2009, 27(1):31–40.

19. Schene AH, van Wijngaarden B, Koeter MWJ. Involvement evaluation questionnaire-European version. Academic Medical Center, Amsterdam, The Netherlands: Department of Psychiatry, 2001.

20. Gawande A. *Being mortal: medicine and what matters in the end*. Metropolitan Books, 2014.

# EPILOGUE

Christopher Dowrick

We hope that you have found this book useful, in providing practical, evidence-based advice on how to assess, manage and relieve your patients' mental health problems. We will be pleased to receive feedback from you, not only on what you have found most helpful, but also how we might improve the content in future editions. If you wish to do so, you may contact us on mhconsult@wonca.net.

The WONCA Working Party on Mental Health (WWPMH) continues to develop new guidance on mental health care for family doctors. As well as the topics covered in this book, we are planning to provide further guidance for family doctors on the management of alcohol and drug-related harms and on interventions for early years problems. These will be posted on the WWPMH pages of the WONCA website: www.wonca.net.

The attention of family doctors is usually, and reasonably, on the individual patient and their family and carers. However, we also need to be aware of the substantial impact on mental health of socio-economic factors, such as poverty, unemployment and discrimination, and humanitarian catastrophes related to climate change or political conflict. As family doctors, we are in a strong position to bring our influence to bear as advocates for health promotion and broader structural change. WWPMH is planning to issue further guidance on effective responses to mental health problems generated by humanitarian emergencies. We are also committed to encouraging and training young family doctors in the advocacy skills needed to effect policy and system change.

Eric Cassel reminds us that our primary obligation in medicine is not the cure of disease, but the relief of suffering.[1] I agree profoundly with Cassel, but wish to add an additional key element to our roles as family doctors: not only acknowledging suffering, but also offering hope.[2] We are in a unique and privileged position to do so, for those many patients who consult us in deep emotional distress.

Bearing witness to our patients' suffering, giving them a sense of being understood and accepted, is the first essential step towards hope. It is my hope and expectation that the advice offered in this book will encourage you and your patients to take many further steps on your journeys towards mental health and wellbeing.

# References

1. Cassel EJ. The nature of suffering and the goals of medicine. *N Engl J Med*. 1982, 306: 639–645.
2. Dowrick C. Suffering and hope: 3rd Helen Lester memorial lecture. *BJGP Open*. 2017: BJGP-2016-0584.

# Answers to multiple choice questions

Chapter 1: 1b, 2d, 3b, 4a, 5c

Chapter 2: 1b, 2c, 3d, 4d, 5d

Chapter 3: 1d, 2c, 3d, 4a

Chapter 4: 1d, 2b, 3d, 4a, 5b

Chapter 5: 1c, 2b, 3c, 4b, 5b

Chapter 7: 1b, 2a, 3c, 4d, 5d

Chapter 8: 1f, 2b & c, 3b & c

Chapter 9: 1b, 2d, 3c, 4a

# Index

Index